KU-308-435

DATE DUE

		.
		PRINTED IN U.S.A.

Content Strategist: Mairi McCubbin
Content Development Specialist: Carole McMurray
Project Manager: Srividhya Vidhyashankar
Designer/Design Direction: Miles Hitchen

The Midwife's Pocket Formulary

Third edition

Liz Davey BSc (Hons) Midwifery, PGDipEd, MA, RGN, RM, DPSM

Senior Lecturer in Midwifery, Bournemouth University, Dorset, UK

Debbee Houghton BSc (Hons) Midwifery Practice, PGDipEd, MAHSCEd RGN, RM, DPSN

Senior Lecturer in Midwifery, Bournemouth University, Dorset, UK

CHURCHILL LIVINGSTONE

ELSEVIER

Edinburgh London New York Oxford Philadelphia St Louis Sydney Toronto 2013

CHURCHILL LIVINGSTONE

ELSEVIER

First edition 1997
Second edition 2004
Third edition 2013
    Reprinted 2013

ISBN 978-0-7020-4347-5

British Library Cataloguing in Publication Data

A catalogue record for this book is available from the British Library

Library of Congress Cataloging in Publication Data

A catalog record for this book is available from the Library of Congress

Notices

Knowledge and best practice in this field are constantly changing. As new research and experience broaden our understanding, changes in research methods, professional practices, or medical treatment may become necessary.

Practitioners and researchers must always rely on their own experience and knowledge in evaluating and using any information, methods, compounds, or experiments described herein. In using such information or methods they should be mindful of their own safety and the safety of others, including parties for whom they have a professional responsibility.

With respect to any drug or pharmaceutical products identified, readers are advised to check the most current information provided (i) on procedures featured or (ii) by the manufacturer of each product to be administered, to verify the recommended dose or formula, the method and duration of administration, and contraindications. It is the responsibility of practitioners, relying on their own experience and knowledge of their patients, to make diagnoses, to determine dosages and the best treatment for each individual patient, and to take all appropriate safety precautions.

To the fullest extent of the law, neither the Publisher nor the authors, contributors, or editors, assume any liability for any injury and/or damage to persons or property as a matter of products liability, negligence or otherwise, or from any use or operation of any methods, products, instructions, or ideas contained in the material herein.

Printed in China

Contents

Introduction

In contemporary midwifery practice, the midwife is required to provide a range of professional competencies and clinical skills in order to promote safe childbirth for women. One of these competencies is medicines management, and midwives and students are required to have an understanding of the range of medicines used within their sphere of practice.

The Nursing and Midwifery Council (NMC) publications (NMC 2004 and 2007) aim to provide structure and clear guidance for the midwifery profession for all aspects of care, including the administration of medications, and directs the professional to use evidence to guide their monitoring and evaluation of medicines in the overall care plan. Within undergraduate education, essential skills relating to medicines are integral to the curriculum, ensuring competence at the point of professional registration.

The aim of this book is to provide a reference text and to guide clinical practice. The student should be aware of:

- the student's role in medicine management
- medicines legislation
- the legal requirements of midwives' exemptions
- the differences and legal requirements between PSDs and PGDs
- the midwives' supply order
- the drug schedules and legal requirements, e.g. controlled drugs
- basic pharmacological principles – pharmacokinetics, pharmacodynamics, pharmacotherapeutics and pharmaceuticals (see Glossary).

Legal Classification of Medicines

The legal controls on the retail sale or supply of medicines are set out in the Medicines Act 1968 and The Human Medicines

Regulations 2012. Medicines are classified into three categories: Prescription-Only Medicine (POM), Pharmacy (P) or General Sale List (GSL). Each category is subject to a number of controls that apply to medicines sold or supplied by retail, or any other form of supply.

Prescription-Only Medicine (POM) – Section 58 of the Medicines Act 1968 Sections 214-219 of The Human Medicines Regulations 2012:

These medicines may be sold or supplied only from a registered pharmacy and in accordance with a prescription issued by an appropriate practitioner (a doctor, dentist, independent (nurse) prescriber, pharmacist independent prescriber or supplementary prescriber) (NMC 2011).

Pharmacy (P) – Section 52 of the Medicines Act 1968 See also Section 220 of The Human Medicines Regulations 2012:

Pharmacy medicines do not require a prescription and may be sold or supplied only in a registered pharmacy by or under the supervision of a pharmacist. The package gives information on dosage (NMC 2011).

General Sale List (GSL) – Section 53 of the Medicines Act 1968 See also Sections 221-222 of The Human Medicines Regulation 2012:

These drugs are those that can be sold with reasonable safety without the supervision of a pharmacist, for example in a supermarket. However, they can be sold only from lockable premises and in the original manufacturers' packs (NMC 2011).

Medicines Unlicensed in the UK

Separate and additional national controls apply to the supply of a medicine that is not licensed for marketing within the UK. Such medicines cannot be advertised. A doctor can prescribe only where the patient has a special need that a licensed medicine cannot meet or where an appropriate licensed medicine is not available.

Midwives' Exemptions

Midwives at the point of registration can supply and/or administer, on their own initiative, any of the substances that are specified in medicines legislation under the midwives' exemptions, provided this is in the course of their professional midwifery practice. In addition they may do so without a prescription, for example a Patient-Specific Direction (PSD) from a medical practitioner or a Patient Group Direction (PGD), provided they have met the requirements attached to the exemption. If a medicine is not included in the midwives' exemptions then a prescription, PSD or a PGD is required (NMC 2011).

Administration of medicines on midwives; exemptions by student midwives

The amended NMC circular (NMC 2011) 'allows student midwives to administer medicines on the midwives exemptions list, except controlled drugs, under the direct supervision of a midwife'. This midwife must be a 'sign-off mentor' and have visual contact throughout the whole administration process by the student midwife. Further, students can 'participate in the checking and preparations of controlled drugs' but not administer them, again under direct supervision of the registrant.

References

Nursing and Midwifery Council (NMC), 2008. The Code: Standards of Conduct, Performance and Ethics for Nurses and Midwives. NMC, London.

Nursing and Midwifery Council (NMC), 2007. updated 2010 Standards for Medicines Management. NMC, London.

Nursing and Midwifery Council (NMC), 2007. NMC Circular 7/2007, 20 March 2007. NMC, London. Available: http://www.nmc-uk.org/Documents/Circulars/2007circulars/NMCcircular07_2007.pdf [accessed 26 March 2012].

Nursing and Midwifery Council (NMC), 2011. NMC Circular 07/2011. 17 June 2011. NMC, London. Available: http://www.nmc-uk.org/Documents/Circulars/2011Circulars/nmcCircular07-2011-Midwives-Exemptions.pdf: Appendix: http://www.nmc-uk.org/Documents/Circulars/2011Circulars/nmcCircular07-2011_Midwives-Exemptions-Annexes.pdf [accessed 30 March 2011].

The Human Medicines Regulations 2012. Available: http://www.legislation.gov.uk/uksi/2012/1916 [accessed 17 January 2013].

The Medicines Act 1968. Available: http://www.legislation.gov.uk/ukpga/1968/67 [accessed 26 March 2012].

Abbreviations

b.d.	*bis die* – twice a day	
t.d.s.	*ter die sumendus* – three times a day	
q.d.s.	*quatre die sumendus* – four times a day	
nocte	at night	
stat	immediately	
p.r.n.	*pro re nata* – as the need arises	
hrly	hourly	
IM	intramuscular – of injections	
IV	intravenous	
IVI	intravenous infusion	
P.O.	per os – by mouth	
P.R.	per rectum – rectally	
P.V.	per vaginam – vaginally	
S.C.	subcutaneous – of injections	
mcg	microgram	
mg	milligram	
g	gram	
kg	kilogram	
mL	millilitre	
L	litre	
ACE	Angiotensin converting enzyme	
ADHD	Attention-deficit/hyperactivity disorder	
APTT	Activated partial prothrombin time – used to monitor clotting when anticoagulant used is heparin	
ARM	Artificial rupture of membranes	
BNF	***British National Formulary*** – information for healthcare professionals from an authoritative and practical focus that is regularly updated in published and online format: Available: http://bnf.org/bnf/index.htm	

CD	Controlled drug
CHM	Commission on Human Medicines
CNS	Central nervous system
CPR	Cardiopulmonary resuscitation
DCT	Direct Coombes test
DVT	Deep vein thrombosis
eMC	***electronic Medicines Compendium*** – information about UK-licensed medicines. Available: http://www.medicines.org.uk/emc/
GABA	Gamma-aminobutyric acid – a deficiency of this inhibitory neurotransmitter may cause excessive responses to excitatory factors and may play a part in the initiation of abnormal discharge, and ultimately convulsions
GI	Gastrointestinal
GSL	General Sales List
GTN	Glyceryl trinitrate
HBIg	Hepatitis B immunoglobulin
HBsAg	Hepatitis B surface antigen
HDN	Haemorrhagic disease of the newborn
HIV	Human immunodeficiency virus
INR	International normalized ratio – usually used to monitor prothrombin time when anticoagulant used is warfarin
IUCD	Intrauterine contraceptive device
IUD	Intrauterine death
LMWH	Low molecular weight heparin
LSCS	Lower-segment caesarean section
MHRA	Medicines and Healthcare products Regulatory Agency
MAOI	Monoamine oxidase inhibitor – a drug that prevents the breakdown of serotonin, leading to an increase in mental and physical activity

MMR	Measles, mumps and rubella (vaccine)
MRP	Manual removal of placenta
MRSA	Methicillin-resistant *Staphylococcus aureus*
NICE	National Institute of Health and Clinical Excellence
NSAID	Non-steroidal anti-inflammatory drug – a drug that inhibits the production of prostaglandins and that has antipyretic, anti-inflammatory and analgesic properties
OCP	Oral contraceptive pill
P	Pharmacy-Only Medicine
PDA	Patient ductus arteriosus
PE	Pulmonary embolus
PGD	**Patient Group Direction** is signed by a doctor and agreed by a pharmacist, which then acts as a direction to a nurse to supply and/or administer prescription-only medicines (POMs) to patients using their own assessment of patient need, without necessarily referring back to a doctor for an individual prescription.
PIL	Patient information leaflet, or PL – package leaflet
PND	Postnatal depression
PPH	Postpartum haemorrhage
PPHN	Persistent pulmonary hypertension in the newborn
POM	Prescription-only medicine
POP	Progestogen-only pill
PSD	**Patient-Specific Direction** is the traditional written instruction, from a doctor, dentist, nurse, midwife or pharmacist, independent prescriber for medicines to be prescribed to a named patient
PT	Prothrombin time
RDS	Respiratory distress syndrome
SLE	Systemic lupus erythematosus

SPC — Summary of product characteristics – written by pharmaceutical companies based on research and product knowledge. These are approved by UK and European licensing agencies after checking

SRM — Spontaneous rupture of membranes

SSRI — Selective serotonin reuptake inhibitor – these drugs inhibit the reuptake of serotonin at nerve terminals, leading to inhibition of excitatory impulses and subsequent overload, and are used in conditions such as depression, anxiety and panic disorders

TCA — Tricyclic antidepressants – complex action but thought to inhibit the uptake and reuptake of serotonin and noradrenaline (norepinephrine)

UFH — Unfractionated heparin

URTI — Upper respiratory tract infection

UTI — Urinary tract infection

VZV — Varicella-zoster virus

Glossary of Terms

Anticholinergic – a drug that inhibits the effects of acetylcholine, a chemical transmitter released by some nerve endings at the synapse between one neuron and another, or the nerve endings and the effector organ. It supplies the lower motor neurons and parasympathetic nerves. Anticholinergic drugs relax smooth muscle, are antispasmodics, and inhibit secretory responses and vomiting

Antimuscarinic – a synthetic anticholinergic drug; the opposite of a muscarinic drug

Extrapyramidal – affecting the nerve tracts outside the pyramidal (spinal) tract

Mendelson syndrome – acid aspiration in obstetric women during delivery, usually associated with general anaesthesia

Muscarinic – causes sympathetic symptoms, i.e. the actions of acetylcholine on the nerve endings and the sympathetic nerves; for example, increases salivation, bronchial secretions, gastrointestinal activity

Myasthenia gravis – an extreme form of muscle weakness, thought to be related to the rapid destruction of acetylcholine at neurotransmitter junctions

Pharmaceutical drug – a medicine, medication, or medicant or chemical substance used in diagnosis, treatment or prevention of disease

Pharmcokinetics – how the body handles the medication

Pharmacodynamics – actions of the medication on the body

Pharmacotherapeutics – the effect of the medication on the body

Wernicke's encephalopathy – a neurological condition due to vitamin B1 (thiamine) deficiency. In relation to midwifery care it may be seen in women with severe hyperemesis

1

Anaesthesia

These drugs depress part of the central nervous system, causing the loss of sensation in a part of or in the whole of the body. There are two main groups, inhalational and intravenous.

These drugs are the specialty of an anaesthetist, although midwives do use certain ones, e.g. 50% nitrous oxide and 50% oxygen via Entonox™ apparatus (or piped supply), or local agents such as lidocaine for perineal infiltration and bupivacaine for epidural top-ups. This chapter explores the anaesthetics used by midwives and not those administered by anaesthetists alone. It is also of note that in the 2006–2008 Saving Mother's Lives, the 8th Report of the Confidential Enquiries into Maternal Deaths in the United Kingdom (Centre for Maternal and Child Enquiries, 2011), anaesthesia was directly responsible for seven deaths (3%), although anaesthesia contributed to 18 (a considerable number), several where the outcome was compromised by the anaesthetic management and provision of high-dependency care.

Midwives need to be aware of the action of anaesthetics, and maternity units need to provide recovery areas for patients having a caesarean section and high-risk clients.

The student should be aware of:

- the difference between analgesia and anaesthesia
- the difference between local, regional and general anaesthesia
- the physiology and pathophysiology of the perception of pain

- the physiological principles underpinning epidural anaesthesia
- problems that occur with obstetrical anaesthesia, i.e. the effects of progesterone on the mother, the presence of two patients rather than one, the pressure of the gravid uterus
- updated resuscitation techniques
- how to apply cricoid pressure if requested to in an emergency.

BP
Nitrous oxide

Proprietary
Entonox™ (BOC Healthcare)

Group
Anaesthetic, inhalational

Uses/indications
Analgesia during labour

Type of drug
POM, midwives' exemptions or PGD

Presentation
Colourless gas with slightly sweet odour in cylinders – blue with blue and white quarters at the valve end and labelled Entonox
Cylinders should be: stored under cover; not stored near stocks of combustible materials
F size cylinders and larger should be stored vertically. D size cylinders and smaller may be stored horizontally ensure cylinders are maintained at a temperature above 10°C for at least 24 h before use to ensure the gases are mixed correctly. Care needed when handling and using gas-filled cylinders, including transportation – cylinders should be separate from the driver area, securely held, and emergency procedures known to the driver. Use of a hazard warning label is essential

Dosage
50% nitrous oxide:50% oxygen, self-administered via mask or Entonox™ equipment

Route of admin
Inhalational

Contraindications
Pneumothorax, facial or jaw injuries, diving accidents, overt drunkenness

Side effects
Drowsiness, nausea, vomiting

Interactions
None specific, but BNF (2011) indicates that it may be appropriate to consider that nitrous oxide enhances the effect of other anaesthetics or analgesics, and is similar in action to a general anaesthetic. Relevant interactions to obstetrics are that:

Anxiolytics and hypnotics – enhances the sedative effect
Methyldopa – increases the hypotensive effect

Pharmacodynamic properties
Medical gas – colourless
Oxygen – odourless and present in the atmosphere at 21%; nitrous oxide – sweet smelling and potent analgesic from endorphin release when at 25% concentration, but weak anaesthetic

Fetal risk
Can depress neonatal respiration (BNF 2011). It is also of note that it may increase the risk of spontaneous abortion and low birthweight in female workers where levels of exposure are raised, i.e. operating theatres, labour wards

Breastfeeding
No data available on controlled studies during breastfeeding

BP
Lidocaine hydrochloride

Proprietary
Lidocaine hydrochloride 1% and 2% (Goldshield Group Ltd)

Group
Local anaesthetic

Uses/indications
Perineal infiltration – prior to episiotomy or suturing, **or for nerve blocks**
Emergency use, e.g. cardiac arrest – see Chapter 25 for indications, usage, and dosage

Type of drug
POM, midwives' exemptions or PGD

Presentation
Glass or polypropylene ampoules 2, 5, 10 or 20 mL, with strength, 1% or 2%, indicated on the ampoule

Dosage
As per unit protocol, lowest concentration and smallest dose producing the required effect

Route of admin
Injection

Contraindications
Hypersensitivity and profound hypovolaemia

Side effects
Hypotension, bradycardia, hypersensitivity can lead to anaphylaxis, although this is rare; also inadvertent IV injection can lead to central nervous system excitatory response and then drowsiness, convulsions and respiratory arrest

Interactions
(Less likely when used topically)

Anaesthetics – action of suxamethonium is prolonged, bupivacaine increases the risk of myocardial depression

Antacids – cimetidine increases the plasma concentration absorption of lidocaine and can increase the risk of toxicity

Antipsychotics – increased risk of toxicity with myelosuppressive drugs

β-blockers – increased risk of myocardial depression with propranolol

Pharmacodynamic properties
Stabilizes the neuronal membrane and prevents the initiation and conduction of nerve impulses, causing profound anaesthesia of the membranes and lubrication that reduces friction. Effective in 5 min and lasts for 20–30 min

Fetal risk
Crosses placental barriers and can therefore cause after large doses neonatal respiratory depression, hypertonia, bradycardia after paracervical block, or accidental direct injection during infiltration of the perineum prior to episiotomy

Breastfeeding
Small amounts are secreted into breast milk, thus manufacturers indicate caution if used in nursing mothers

---

BP
Bupivacaine hydrochloride

Proprietary
Marcain® 0.125% and 0.5% w/v (AstraZeneca UK Ltd)
Marcain Heavy® 0.5% w/v (AstraZeneca UK Ltd)

Group
Local anaesthetic

Continued

Uses/indications
Epidural anaesthesia, spinal anaesthesia

Type of drug
POM

Presentation
Polypropylene ampoules (Steripacks) of differing percentages

Dosage
As prescribed by the anaesthetist

Route of admin
Intrathecal injection

Contraindications
Hypovolaemia, hypotension, pyrexia in labour, pyogenic infection of the skin at or adjacent to the lumbar site, coagulation disorders or ongoing coagulation treatment, known hypersensitivity to local anaesthetics such as lidocaine, meningitis, hypovolae-mic shock, intracranial haemorrhage, cardiogenic shock, low levels of platelets

Side effects
Anaphylaxis, maternal hypotension, bradycardia – preloading with crystalloids required – persistent or profound symptoms can be reversed with ephedrine 10–15 mg IV, myocardial depression and seizures if given IV, may cause maternal pyrexia and some diminishing of uterine contractions, post-lumbar headache. A high block causes respiratory embarrass-ment, arrest and paralysis, neurological problems include paraesthesia, motor weakness and loss of sphincter control; accidental IV injection – causes numbness of the tongue, tinnitus, light-headedness, dizziness and tremors, followed by drowsiness, convulsions and cardiac disorders, and requires the attendance of skilled anaesthetic help

Interactions
Antiarrhythmics – increased myocardial depression

Pharmacodynamic properties
Marcain Heavy® – local anaesthetic of the amide type
that causes moderate relaxation of lower extremities
and a motor blockade of abdominal muscles
Marcain (bupivacaine) – as above, but analgesia
without the motor blockade

Fetal risk
Reportedly bradycardia, respiratory depression, fetal
hypothermia; toxicity in animal studies indicates
avoidance in early pregnancy, but manufacturers
suggest there is no evidence of untoward effects

Breastfeeding
Excreted in small amounts but no risk from therapeutic
doses

BP
Lidocaine hydrochloride 2.5% and Prilocaine 2.5%

Proprietary
Emla 5% Cream™ (AstraZeneca UK Ltd)

Group
Anaesthetic – local

Uses/indications
Anaesthesia prior to venepuncture, surface analgesia

Type of drug
POM

Presentation
White soft cream

Dosage
Thick layer 1–5 h prior to procedure under occlusive
dressing

Route of admin
Topical

Continued

Contraindications
Dermatitis at site, mucous membrane, wounds or hypersensitivity to active constituents

Side effects
Transient paleness, redness and oedema have been reported

Interactions
As for lidocaine, but unlikely

Pharmacodynamic properties
Provides dermal analgesia, depending on application time and dose, by causing transient local vasoconstriction or vasodilation at the treated area

Fetal risk
Crosses the placental barrier, but no ill effects have been reported

Breastfeeding
Excreted in breast milk in small amounts but considered safe

BP
Lidocaine hydrochloride 2% and Chlorhexidine gluconate 0.25%

Proprietary
Instillagel® (CliniMed)

Group
Anaesthetic – local (surface anaesthesia)

Uses/indications
anaesthesia of the urethra prior to catheterization, or topical application to mucous membranes, i.e. the perineum

Type of drug
POM

Presentation
Ampoules of gel or in accordion gel pack

Dosage
5–10 mL intraurethrally to fill urethra

Route of admin
Topical/intraurethral

Contraindications
Hypersensitivity to lidocaine. Trauma to the urethra can cause increased systemic absorption

Side effects
As for lidocaine but fewer, as topically applied

Interactions
As for lidocaine, but unlikely

Pharmacodynamic properties
Stabilizes the neuronal membrane and prevents the initiation and conduction of nerve impulses, causing profound anaesthesia of the membranes and lubrication that reduces friction. Effective in 5 min and lasts for 20–30 min

Fetal risk
No evidence of harm but avoid in early pregnancy

Breastfeeding
No evidence of risk

References and Recommended Reading

Bartholomew, C., Yerby, M., 2011. Pain, labour and women's choice of pain relief. In: Macdonald, S., Magill-Cuerden, J. (Eds.), Mayes' Midwifery, fourteenth ed. Baillière Tindall/Elsevier, Edinburgh, pp. 521–534.

Baxter, K., 2011. Stockley's Drug Interaction Companion. Pharmaceutical Press, London.

Briggs, G., Freeman, R., Yaffe, S., 2008. Drugs in Pregnancy and Lactation: A Reference Guide to Fetal and Neonatal Risk, eighth ed. Lippincott Williams and Wilkins, Philadelphia.

Bubimschi, C., Weiner, C., 2010. Medication. In: James, D.K., Steer, P.J., Weiner, C.P., Gonik, B. (Eds.), High Risk Pregnancy: Management Options, fourth ed. Elsevier Saunders, London, pp. 579–598.

Hofmeyr, G.J., Neilson, J.P., Alfreirevic, Z., Crowther, C., Duley, L., Gulmezoglu, M., Gyte, G.M., Hodnett, E.D. 2008. Pregnancy and Childbirth – a Cochrane Pocketbook. Wiley Cochrane Series, London

Instillagel® (Lidocaine hydrochloride 2% and Chlorhexidine gluconate 0.25%), Clinimed, updated in BNF 62, 2011.

Joint Formulary Committee, 2011. British National Formulary (BNF) 62. Pharmaceutical Press, London.

Jordan, S., 2010. Pain relief. In: Jordan, S. (Ed.), Pharmacology for Midwives: The Evidence Base for Safe Practice, second ed. Palgrave Macmillan, Basingstoke.

Koren, G., 2007. Medication Safety in Pregnancy and Breastfeeding: The Evidence Based A–Z Clinician's Pocket Guide. McGraw-Hill, New York.

Paediatric Formulary Committee, 2011. BNF for Children 2011–2012. Pharmaceutical Press, London.

Rubin, P.C., Ramsey, M., 2007. Prescribing in Pregnancy, fourth ed. BMJ Books/Blackwell Publishing, Oxford.

Schaefer, C., Peters, P.W.J., Miller, R.K. (Eds.), 2007. Drugs During Pregnancy and Lactation: Treatment Options and Risk Assessment, Academic Press/Elsevier, London.

SPC from BOC gases, Entonox™, BOC Healthcare updated 9/2/10.

SPC from the eMC, Emla® Cream, AstraZeneca UK Ltd, updated on the eMC 15/8/11.

SPC from the eMC, Lidocaine Hydrochloride 1% and 2% Goldshield Group Ltd, updated on the eMC 29/9/11 and 12/10/11.

SPC from the eMC, Marcain® Heavy, AstraZeneca UK Ltd, updated on the eMC 19/11/10.

SPC from the eMC, Marcain® Polyamp Steripack 0.5%, Goldshield Healthcare Ltd, updated on the eMC 1/12/10.

Tsen, L.C., 2010. Neuroxial analgesia and anaesthesia in pregnancy. In: James, D.K., Steer, P.J., Weiner, C.P., Gonik, B. (Eds.), High Risk Pregnancy: Management Options, fourth ed. Elsevier Saunders, London, pp. 1211–1230.

Varner, R.G., 1993. Mechanisms of regurgitation and its prevention with cricoid pressure. International Journal of Obstetrical Anaesthesia 2, 207–215.

Volans, G., Wiseman, H., 2012. Drugs Handbook 2012–2013, thirtythird ed. Palgrave Macmillan, Basingstoke.

Further Reading

Centre for Maternal and Child Enquiries 2011 Saving Mothers' Lives, Reviewing Maternal Deaths to Make Motherhood Safer: 2006–2008. The 8th Report of the Confidential Enquiries into Maternal Deaths in the United Kingdom. Available http://www.oaa-anaes.ac.uk/assets/_managed/editor/File/Reports/2006-2008%20CEMD.pdf [accessed 2 March 2012].

Hofmeyr, G.J., Neilson, J.P., Alfreirevic, Z., Crowther, C., Duley, L., Gulmezoglu, M., Gyte, G.M., Hodnett, E.D. 2008. Pregnancy and Childbirth – a Cochrane Pocketbook. Wiley Cochrane Series, London.

Yentis, S., May, A., Malhatra, S., 2007. Analgesia, Anaesthesia and Pregnancy – A, Practical Guide, second ed. Cambridge University Press, Cambridge.

2

Analgesics

These preparations are used to relieve pain without causing unconsciousness or lack of all nervous sensation in a particular area. It is important to become familiar with pain theories and to use the body's natural analgesics to their optimum effect, as well as using chemical preparations.

The student should be aware of:

- pain theories, especially the 'gate theory' of Melzack and Wall (1964)
- the difference between anaesthesia and analgesia
- the accumulative effect of many analgesics, which can lead to intentional or accidental overdose
- the different combinations of separate analgesic compounds
- the possibility of addiction to analgesics
- neonatal sequelae to maternal analgesia
- the appropriateness of the analgesic compound to the complaint.

BP
Paracetamol (Acetaminophen)

Proprietary
Paracetamol (Actavis UK Ltd) (refer to BNF for manufacturers and advice on trade names)
Calpol® infant suspension (McNeil Products Ltd; Pinewood Healthcare) (refer to BNF for manufacturers and advice on trade names)

Group
Analgesic, non-opioid

Uses/indications
Mild to moderate pain, headache, rheumatic pain, pyrexia

Type of drug
POM, GSL (sold to the public in packs of no more than 16 tablets; pharmacists may dispense up to 32 tablets)

Presentation
Tablets, oral suspension, dispersible tablets, suppositories

Dosage
Adult: oral: 500 mg–1 g 4–6-hrly (max 4 g daily); P.R.: 0.5–1 g q.d.s.
Paediatric: oral – dose calculated on 10 mg per kg body weight

Route of admin
Oral, P.R.

Contraindications
Hypersensitivity, hepatic and renal disease, alcohol dependence

Side effects
Rare, blood disorders, rashes, overdose causes liver damage, pancreatitis with prolonged use

Interactions
Anticoagulants – with prolonged use seems to enhance effect of warfarin
Cholestyramine – reduces the absorption of paracetamol
Metaclopromide – enhances the effect of paracetamol

Pharmacodynamic properties
Antipyretic, peripherally acting analgesic

Fetal risk
Epidemiological studies in human pregnancy show no ill effects

Continued

Breastfeeding
Short courses only – amount secreted too small to be harmful. No controlled study data available and taken by a large number of women with no observed increase in adverse effects on breastfed infants, therefore considered safe

BP
Aspirin (Acetylsalicylic acid)

Proprietary
Aspirin (Actavis UK Ltd)
(Various generic manufacturers; see BNF for advice)

Group
Analgesic, non-opioid, NSAID

Uses/indications
Mild to moderate pain, including headache, neuralgia, rheumatic pain, transient musculoskeletal pain, pyrexia

Type of drug
GSL (sold to the public in packs of no more than 16 tablets; pharmacists may dispense up to 32 capsules/ tablets), POM

Presentation
Tablets, some dispersible, suppositories

Dosage
300–900 mg 4–6-hrly to a max 4 g daily

Route of admin
Oral, P.R.

Contraindications
Hypersensitivity, clotting disorders, haemophilia, asthma, angio-oedema, urticaria, rhinitis, impaired renal or hepatic function, dehydration, gastric ulceration, pregnancy, unless in very low doses on obstetrician's orders

Side effects
Increased bleeding time, leading to haemorrhage, i.e. antepartum, intrapartum, postpartum, delayed onset and duration of labour (low doses are not harmful) mild and infrequent, gastric irritation/ulceration, hypersensitivity, bronchospasm and skin reactions in hypersensitive patients, haematuria, nervousness, dizziness, tinnitus, insomnia, rash

Interactions
Alcohol – enhanced effect on the gut
Antacids – increased alkalinity of urine
Analgesics – concomitant admin increases side effects
Anticoagulants – increased risk of haemorrhage (potentiates antiplatelet effect)
Antiepileptics – enhanced effect of phenytoin and valproate
Corticosteroids – enhances the risk of gastrointestinal bleeding and ulceration
Metoclopramide – increases rate of absorption and therefore increased effects of aspirin

Pharmacodynamic properties
Aspirin is an analgesic, antipyretic, anti-inflammatory that inhibits the synthesis of prostaglandins

Fetal risk
Low-dose aspirin is not thought to have harmful effects; in high doses closure of PDA in utero, persistent pulmonary hypertension, possible reduction in the amount of amniotic fluid (Bubimschi and Weiner, 2010) not recommended after 34 weeks' gestation, kernic-terus in jaundiced neonates; is also reported to be linked with fetal growth deficiency and a purpuric rash in neonates, with depression of the platelet function

Breastfeeding
Potentially Reye's syndrome (under 16s specifically), regular high doses could cause impairment of platelet function and hypoprothrombinaemia if neonatal vitamin K stores are low

BP
Codeine phosphate

Proprietary
Codeine phosphate (Actavis UK Ltd)
Codeine phosphate (non-proprietary, see BNF for details)

Group
Analgesic, opioid – morphine salt

Uses/indications
Mild to moderate pain, cough suppressant

Type of drug
POM, (CD – injection)

Presentation
Tablets, syrup, ampoules (CD)

Dosage
Oral: 30–60 mg 4-hrly (max 240 mg daily); IM: 30–60 mg 4 hrly

Route of admin
Oral, IM

Contraindications
As for morphine, raised intracranial pressure

Side effects
Constipation, nausea, sedation, respiratory depression, especially cough reflex, dependence. In labour – maternal gastric stasis and increased risk of inhalation pneumonia

Interactions
As for diamorphine

Pharmacodynamic properties
Codeine is a narcotic analgesic that acts via the central nervous system

Fetal risk
First trimester: inguinal hernias, cardiac, circulatory and
respiratory system defects, cleft lip and palate, although
not according to Bubimschi and Weiner (2010)
second trimester: alimentary tract defects
labour: neonatal respiratory depression and withdrawal

Breastfeeding
Amount of active metabolites secreted too small to be
harmful and limited data available on breastfeeding
women, where there was no observed increase in
adverse effects on breastfed infants

BP
Co-codaprin

Proprietary
Co-codaprin (non-proprietary, see BNF for details)

Group
Analgesic, aspirin compound (aspirin 400 mg + codeine
phosphate 8 mg)

Uses/indications
Mild to moderate pain

Type of drug
POM

Presentation
Tablets (white)

Dosage
1–2 tablets 4–6-hrly (max 8 daily)

Route of admin
Oral

Contraindications
As for codeine and aspirin

Side effects
As for codeine and aspirin

Interactions
As for codeine and aspirin

Fetal risk
As for codeine and aspirin

Breastfeeding
Codeine is excreted in small amounts. Manufacturers recommend to avoid administration of opioids in breastfeeding; should also be avoided in view of aspirin content, although there are no controlled studies available for breastfeeding women

---

BP
Co-dydramol (Paracetamol 500 mg + Dihydrocodeine 10 mg)

Proprietary
Co-dydramol tablets 10/500 mg (Actavis UK Ltd)

Group
Analgesic, paracetamol and opioid compound

Uses/indications
Mild to moderate pain

Type of drug
POM, GSL

Presentation
Tablets (white)

Dosage
1–2 tablets 4–6-hrly (max 8 daily)

Route of admin
Oral

Contraindications
As for paracetamol and dihydrocodeine

Side effects
As for paracetamol and dihydrocodeine

Interactions
As for paracetamol and dihydrocodeine

Fetal risk
As for dihydrocodeine

Breastfeeding
No controlled study data available for breastfeeding
and the risk of untoward effects in a breastfed infant is a
possibility. The compound is considered safe, as it has
been taken by a large number of women with no
observed increase in adverse effects in infants

BP
Co-proxamol (Paracetamol 325 mg + Dextropropoxyphene 325 mg)

Proprietary
Distalgesic® (Dista Products Ltd) **NB:** No longer licensed
due to safety concerns, but may be prescribed for
patients who find it difficult to change (BNF 62, 2011).

Group
Analgesic, compound of paracetamol and opioid salt

Uses/indications
Mild to moderate pain

Type of drug
POM (CD), GSL

Presentation
Tablets (white marked DG)

Dosage
1–2 tablets 4–6-hrly (max 8 daily)

Route of admin
Oral

Contraindications
Alcohol abuse, hypersensitivity to either of the
constituents, addictive or suicidal clients, hepatic or
renal impairment, concomitant paracetamol usage

Side effects
Dizziness, sedation, nausea, vomiting, constipation,
abdominal pain, headache. NB: *overdose* is complicated
by respiratory depression, heart failure and by hepatic
failure, and *can cause death in 15 minutes*

Interactions
CNS depressant effect of the opioid constituent enhances the effect of CNS depressants, including alcohol
Anticoagulant – effect of warfarin possibly enhanced
Anticonvulsants – altered metabolism; see above
Antidepressants – altered metabolism; see above

Pharmacodynamic properties
A compound analgesic with a non-narcotic (paracetamol) for relief of pain in musculoskeletal conditions and a narcotic (dextropropoxyphene) for relief of visceral pain

Fetal risk
Not established as safe in pregnancy, withdrawal reported in neonates. Potential benefits should outweigh the possible hazards

Breastfeeding
Amount secreted too small to be harmful

BP
Co-codamol (Paracetamol 500 mg + Codeine 8 mg)

Proprietary
Co-codamol (Wockhardt UK Ltd)
– paracetamol 500 mg + codeine 30 mg

Group
Analgesic, paracetamol and opioid compound

Uses/indications
Mild to moderate pain

Type of drug
POM

Presentation
Tablets, capsules, dispersible tablets

Dosage
1–2 tablets or capsules 4-hrly, max 8 daily

Route of admin
Oral

Contraindications
As for paracetamol and codeine

Side effects
As for paracetamol and codeine phosphate

Interactions
As for paracetamol and codeine phosphate

Fetal risk
As for codeine phosphate

Breastfeeding
No controlled study data available for breastfeeding
and the risk of untoward effects in a breastfed infant is a
possibility. The compound is considered safe, as it has
been taken by a large number of women with no
observed increase in adverse effects in infants

BP
Ibuprofen

Proprietary
Brufen® (Abbott Healthcare Products Ltd)
(GSL – Nurofen®, Crookes Healthcare Ltd)
Ibuprofen (non-proprietary, see BNF for details)

Group
Analgesic, non-opioid, NSAID

Uses/indications
Mild to moderate pain, particularly perineal

Type of drug
POM, (GSL)

Presentation
Tablets, syrup, granules

Dosage
1.2–1.8 g daily in 3–4 doses (after food)

Route of admin
Oral

Contraindications
Pregnancy, salicylate hypersensitivity, asthma

Side effects
Gastrointestinal discomfort, diarrhoea, nausea, rash, headache, dizziness

Interactions
As for diclofenac and salicylic acid

Pharmacodynamic properties
Analgesic, anti-inflammatory, antipyretic; this NSAID is thought to act by inhibiting prostaglandin synthesis

Fetal risk
As for salicylic acid, delayed onset and increased duration of labour

Breastfeeding
Limited studies suggest NSAIDs can appear in the breast milk in very low concentrations; manufacturer recommends avoid during breastfeeding

---

BP
Mefenamic acid

Proprietary
Ponstan™ (Chemidex Pharma Ltd)

Group
Analgesic, non-opioid, NSAID

Uses/indications
Mild to moderate pain, postpartum pain, postoperative pain, anti-inflammatory

Type of drug
POM

Presentation
Tablets, capsules

Dosage
500 mg t.d.s. after food

Route of admin
Oral

Contraindications
Hypersensitivity to mefenamic acid, irritable bowel syndrome, peptic/intestinal ulceration, renal or hepatic impairment, asthma or allergic reactions, i.e. rhinitis or urticaria or bronchospasm on administration of NSAIDs

Side effects
Drowsiness, diarrhoea, nausea, rash, thrombocytopenia, haemolytic anaemia or purpuric rash. If these occur withdraw the drug; hypersensitive reaction – bronchospasm, urticaria, nausea, vomiting, abdominal pain, headache, facial oedema, laryngeal oedema, dizziness, abnormal vision, palpitations

Interactions
As for diclofenac, but especially
Anticoagulants – increased effect
Antihypertensives – reduces the hypotensive effect
OVERDOSE – can cause convulsions

Pharmacodynamic properties
A prostaglandin synthesis inhibiting NSAID with anti-inflammatory, antipyretic effects and analgesic properties

Fetal risk
Safety is not established and possibly has same effects as salicylic acid; known effects of NSAIDs on the fetal cardiovascular system (risk of closure of the ductus arteriosus); use in the last trimester of pregnancy is contraindicated

Breastfeeding
Trace amounts may be present in breast milk and transmitted to the infant, therefore manufacturers recommend against use during breastfeeding

Continued

BP
Diclofenac sodium

Proprietary
Voltarol® (Novartis Pharmaceuticals UK Ltd)
diclofenac sodium (non-proprietary, see BNF for
details)

Group
Analgesic, non-opioid, NSAID

Uses/indications
Moderate to severe pain, musculoskeletal pain, used
post LSCS, anti-inflammatory properties

Type of drug
POM, GSL

Presentation
Tablets some dispersible, ampoules, suppositories

Dosage
Oral: 75–150 mg daily in divided doses, preferably after
food (max 150 mg in 24 h)
P.R.: 100 mg 18–24-hrly (max 150 mg in 24 h)
Rarely – deep IM: 75 mg daily (max 2 days)

Route of admin
Oral, P.R., rarely deep IM

Contraindications
Asthma, pregnancy, hypersensitivity to NSAIDs, cardiac,
hepatic or renal impairment, clotting disorders

Side effects
Uterine inertia, delayed onset and increased duration of
labour, increased postpartum blood loss, coagulation
disorders leading to haemorrhage, asthma, bronchospasm, gastric irritability/ulceration, rectal irritation,
headache, dizziness, vertigo, abdominal pain, rash,
purpura, urticaria, drowsiness, disturbances of vision,
loss of sensation, malaise, fatigue and insomnia

Interactions
Analgesics – concomitant admin, causes increased side effects

Antihypertensives – calcium channel blockers; antagonizes hypotensive effects

β-blockers – antagonism of hypotensive effects

Methlydopa – antagonism of the hypotensive effect

Anticoagulants – coumarins – anticoagulant effect is increased

Heparin – increased risk of haemorrhage with IV diclofenac

Antiepileptics – phenytoin – possible enhanced effect

Zidovudine – increased risk of haematological toxicity

Pharmacodynamic properties
NSAID analgesic that inhibits prostaglandin synthesis, with antipyretic properties

Fetal risk
Benefits must outweigh the risk and the lowest possible effective dose should be used; can cause closure of PDA in utero, persistent pulmonary hypertension

Breastfeeding
Amount secreted too small to be harmful and evidence of risk is remote, although there are only a limited number of controlled studies in breastfeeding women

BP
Diamorphine hydrochloride

Proprietary
Diamorphine Hydrochloride Injection (Auralis Ltd)

Group
Analgesic – morphine salt – narcotic

Uses/indications
Moderate to severe pain, i.e. postoperative and labour

Type of drug
POM, CD authorized by PGD and Midwives' Exemptions

Continued

Presentation
Tablets, powder for reconstitution

Dosage
5–10 mg 4-hrly (depending on recipient size)
slow IV injection: 0.25–0.5 of the corresponding IM dose

Route of admin
IM, oral, slow IV injection

Contraindications
Existing respiratory depression, asthma, raised intracranial pressure as it affects papillary responses, phaeochromocytoma – endogenous release of histamines may stimulate catecholamine release

Side effects
Gastric stasis in labour, sedation, nausea, vomiting, respiratory depression, dependence, tachycardia, hypothermia, hallucinations, mood swings, facial flushing, sweating, constipation, dizziness, miosis, confusion, urinary retention, biliary spasm, postural hypotension, vertigo, palpitations, dry mouth, urticaria, pruritus, raised intracranial pressure and rarely circulatory depression

Interactions
Non-specific to diamorphine but characteristic of opioids
Alcohol – enhances the sedative effect, increases hypotension
Analgesics – enhanced effects
Antidepressants – avoid concurrent administration of MAOI or administration within 2 weeks of their discontinuation increases the sedative effect of tricyclics
Anxiolytics and hypnotics – enhances the sedative effect
Cimetidine – inhibits metabolism, thereby increasing the plasma concentration of the opioid
Metoclopramide – antagonism of the effect on gastrointestinal activity

Pharmacodynamic properties
Narcotic analgesic acting on the central nervous system (CNS) and smooth muscle. Its predominant action is to depress the CNS, but it has stimulant actions resulting in nausea, vomiting and miosis

Fetal risk
Crosses the placental barrier within 1 h of administration; causes withdrawal symptoms, respiratory depression, meconium aspiration, intrauterine death

Breastfeeding
Therapeutic doses are unlikely to affect the infant, but in dependent mothers secretion into breast milk may cause problems with withdrawal and addiction

---

BP
Morphine sulphate

Proprietary
Oramorph® 10 mg/5 mL (Boehringer Ingelheim Ltd)
Morphine sulphate (Wockhardt UK Ltd)
Morphine sulphate (non-proprietary, see BNF for details)

Group
Analgesic – narcotic

Uses/indications
Postoperative pain, to potentiate epidural anaesthesia, Patient-controlled analgesia systems (PCAS)

Type of drug
POM, P, CD

Presentation
Oral solution, tablets, capsules, suspension, suppositories, ampoules

Continued

Dosage

IM or S.C.: 10–15 mg 4-hrly (depending on patient size, severity of pain, response and tolerance to dosage)

slow IV injection: 0.25–0.5 of IM dose

intrathecal: dosage determined by anaesthetist

PCAS: determined by hospital protocols

oral: rare in obstetrics – refer to BNF, but usually double IM dose; post LSCS usage is increasing, refer to BNF but typically 10–20 mL 3-hrly

P.R.: 15–30 mg 4-hrly

Route of admin

Oral, IM, S.C., P.R., IV, intrathecal

Contraindications

Renal or hepatic impairment, respiratory depression, asthma, raised intracranial pressure (affects papillary responses), phaeochromocytoma

Side effects

As for diamorphine. NB: postoperative patients should be observed closely for delayed or rebound respiratory depression as well as other side effects

Interactions

As for diamorphine

Pharmacodynamic properties

Morphine is a narcotic analgesic obtained from opium; acts on the central nervous system and smooth muscle

Fetal risk

As for diamorphine and pethidine

Breastfeeding

Therapeutic doses unlikely to affect the infant and so considered moderately safe

BP
Fentanyl

Proprietary
Fentanyl citrate (Goldshield Group Ltd)
(Non-proprietary, see BNF for details)

Group
Analgesic, opioid – morphine salt

Uses/indications
Enhancement of anaesthesia, i.e. epidural

Type of drug
CD

Presentation
Prediluted ampoules, premixed solution in polybags of
100 or 200 mL for intrathecal infusion in continuous
epidurals

Dosage
50–200 micrograms (mcg), subsequent doses 50 mcg
p.r.n.

Route of admin
Intrathecal (IM or IV not used in obstetrics)

Contraindications
Caution in existing respiratory depression, myasthenia
gravis, known hypersensitivity to fentanyl or opioids

Side effects
Respiratory depression – can be delayed, apnoea,
transient hypotension, bradycardia, nausea, vomiting,
itching, muscular rigidity, myoclonic movements,
urinary retention. Hypersensitivity can cause
anaphylaxis

Interactions
As for morphine

Continued

Pharmacodynamic properties

A synthetic opiate with 50–100 times the clinical potency of morphine; has a rapid onset but duration of action is short. Its peak effect is at 30 min post dosage; differs from morphine in its short duration of action and its lack of emetic effect

Fetal risk

No evidence of teratogenic or embryotoxic effects, but manufacturers advise avoidance. Crosses the placental barrier and may cause loss of fetal heart variability without fetal hypoxia, respiratory depression or withdrawal symptoms, although these may be less via intrathecal route

Breastfeeding

No controlled study data available. Although it is likely to be present in trace amounts in breast milk and breastfeeding is not recommended for 24 h after administration, there is no evidence of an increased risk of adverse effects in breastfed infants

BP

Dihydrocodeine tartrate

Proprietary
Dihydrocodeine (Goldshield Group UK Ltd)
(non-proprietary, see BNF for details)

Group
Analgesic, opioid – morphine salt

Uses/indications
Moderate to severe pain

Type of drug
POM, (CD – injection)

Presentation
Tablets (white), elixir, ampoules (CD)

Dosage
Oral: 30 mg 4–6-hrly (preferably after food), higher doses cause nausea and vomiting
Deep S.C., IM: 50 mg repeated 4–6-hrly

Route of admin
Oral, IM, deep S.C.

Contraindications
Raised intracranial pressure, respiratory difficulties

Side effects
Constipation, drowsiness, respiratory depression, hypotension, dizziness, dependence; high doses cause nausea and vomiting

Interactions
As for diamorphine

Pharmacodynamic properties
Dihydrocodeine is a semisynthetic narcotic analgesic with a potency between that of morphine and codeine; acts on the opioid receptors in the brain to reduce the patient's perception of pain and improve the psychological reaction to pain by removing associated anxiety

Fetal risk
Little evidence to suggest fetal risk; however, there may be withdrawal symptoms, or respiratory depression in the neonate, and manufacturer advises use only when the benefits outweigh the risks

Breastfeeding
Little evidence to suggest secretion in breast milk, but manufacturers advise avoidance

---

BP
Pethidine hydrochloride

Proprietary
Pethidine Hydrochloride 50 mg/mL (Goldshield Group Ltd)
(Non-proprietary, see BNF for details)

Continued **31**

Group
Analgesic – opioid, alkaloid

Uses/indications
Moderate to severe pain, obstetric analgesia

Type of drug
POM, CD authorized by PGD and Midwives' Exemptions

Presentation
Tablets, ampoules

Dosage
S.C./IM: 25–150 mg 4-hrly
Oral: 50–150 mg 4-hrly
Slow IV injection: 25–50 mg 4-hrly

Route of admin
IM, rarely in obstetrics – oral, S.C., slow IV injection

Contraindications
Existing respiratory depression, renal impairment, pre-existing morphine addiction, compromised fetus

Side effects
Nausea, vomiting, respiratory depression, convulsions after overdose, bradycardia, dependence

Interactions
As for diamorphine
Antacids – cimetidine inhibits metabolism of pethidine

Pharmacodynamic properties
Pethidine binds to opioid receptors and exerts its principal pharmacological actions on the central nervous system where its analgesic and sedative effects are of particular therapeutic value. The respiratory depression produced by pethidine can be antagonized by naloxone and nalorphine. Similar to diamorphine

Fetal risk
Crosses placental barrier within 2 min of administration and present in amniotic fluid in 30 min; bradycardia, respiratory depression, withdrawal symptoms, slow excretion by neonatal liver

Breastfeeding
Depresses suck reflex, as for diamorphine

BP
Meptazinol hydrochloride

Proprietary
Meptid Injection (Almirall Ltd)

Group
Analgesic – opioid of hexahydroazepine group – narcotic

Uses/indications
Moderate to severe pain, i.e. postoperative, renal colic and labour

Type of drug
POM, CD authorized by PGD and Midwives' Exemptions

Presentation
Solution for injection

Dosage
IM 75–150 mg 2–4-hrly (calculated from 2 mg/kg)
slow IV injection 50–100 mg 2–4 hrly as required

Route of admin
IM, slow IV injection

Contraindications
Existing respiratory depression, asthma, raised intracranial pressure as it affects papillary responses, phaeochromocytoma – endogenous release of histamines may stimulate catecholamine release, MAOI medication and for 14 days post discontinuation – central nervous system (CNS) excitation/depression with hypertension/hypotension, acute alcoholism

Continued **33**

Side effects
Gastric stasis in labour, sedation, nausea, vomiting, respiratory depression, dependence, tachycardia, hypothermia, hallucinations, mood swings, facial flushing, sweating, constipation, dizziness, miosis, confusion, urinary retention, biliary spasm, postural hypotension, vertigo, palpitations, dry mouth, urticaria, pruritus, raised intracranial pressure and rarely circulatory depression

Interactions
Non-specific to diamorphine but characteristic of opioids
Alcohol – enhances the sedative effect, increases hypotension
Analgesics – enhanced effects
Antidepressants – avoid concurrent administration of MAOI; administration within 2 weeks of their discontinuation increases the sedative effect of tricyclics
Anxiolytics and hypnotics – enhances the sedative effect
Cimetidine – inhibits metabolism, thereby increasing plasma concentration of the opioid
Metoclopramide – antagonism of the effect on gastrointestinal activity

Pharmacodynamic properties
Centrally acting analgesic of the hexahydroazepine group acting on the CNS and smooth muscle. Predominant action is on opioid receptors, specifically those that have affinity to endogenous opioids (μ δ κ); effects only partly reversed by naloxone

Fetal risk
Crosses the placental barrier within 1 h of administration; respiratory depression, meconium aspiration, intrauterine death

Breastfeeding
Therapeutic doses are unlikely to affect the infant, but manufacturers recommend that benefit should outweigh the risks

BP
Hyoscine butylbromide

Proprietary
Buscopan® (Boehringer Ingelheim Ltd)

Group
Antimuscarinics

Uses/indications
Gastrointestinal smooth muscle spasm, irritable bowel, diverticular disease, dysmenorrhoea

Type of drug
POM, P (GSL – sold to the public provided a single dose does not exceed 20 mg and the daily dose 80 mg; packs are restricted to 240 mg max)

Presentation
Tablets, ampoules

Dosage
Oral: 20 mg q.d.s.
IM, IV injection: 20 mg repeated after 30 min if required

Route of admin
Oral, IM, IV injection

Contraindications
Myasthenia gravis, paralytic ileus

Side effects
Constipation, transient bradycardia followed by tachycardia, palpitations, arrhythmias, urinary urgency and retention, photophobia, dry mouth, flushing and skin dryness; rarely – nausea, vomiting, giddiness, confusion

Interactions
Alcohol – enhances sedative effect of hyoscine
Antidepressants – tricyclics have increased side effects
Antihistamines – increase the antimuscarinic side effects
MAOIs – increased antimuscarinic effects
Phenothiazines – chlorpromazine increases the antimuscarinic side effects

Pharmacodynamic properties

Antispasmodic agent that relaxes the smooth muscle of the organs of the abdominal and pelvic cavities, and acts on the intramural parasympathetic ganglia of these organs

Fetal risk

Animal studies show teratogenicity, but there are no controlled studies in pregnant women. Not recommended by manufacturer unless benefits outweigh the risks

Breastfeeding

Not recommended by manufacturer, but considered moderately safe as there are no observed increases in adverse effects in breastfed infants

References and Recommended Reading

Baxter, K., 2011. Stockley's Drug Interaction Companion. Pharmaceutical Press, London.

Briggs, G., Freeman, R., Yaffe, S., 2008. Drugs in Pregnancy and Lactation: A Reference Guide to Fetal and Neonatal Risk, eighth ed. Lippincott Williams and Wilkins, Philadelphia.

Bubimschi, C., Weiner, C., 2010. Medication. In: James, D.K., Steer, P.J., Weiner, C.P., Gonik, B. (Eds.), High Risk Pregnancy: Management Options, fourth ed. Elsevier Saunders, London, pp. 579–598.

Griffiths, R., 2010. Law, medicines and the midwife. In: Jordan, S. (Ed.), Pharmacology for Midwives: The Evidence Base for Safe Practice, second ed. Palgrave Macmillan, Basingstoke, pp. 62–74.

Hofmeyr, G.J., Neilson, J.P., Alfrirevic, Z., Crowther, C., Duley, L., Gulmezoglu, M., Gyte, G.M., Hodnett, E.D. 2008. Pregnancy and Childbirth – A Cochrane Pocketbook. Wiley Cochrane Series, London.

Joint Formulary Committee, 2011. British National Formulary (BNF) 62. Pharmaceutical Press, London.

Jordan, S., 2010. Pain relief. In: Jordan, S. (Ed.), Pharmacology for Midwives: The Evidence Base for Safe Practice, second ed. Palgrave Macmillan, Basingstoke, pp. 77–130.

Koren, G., 2007. Medication Safety in Pregnancy and Breastfeeding: The Evidence Based A–Z Clinician's Pocket Guide. McGraw-Hill, New York.

Rubin, P.C., Ramsey, M., 2007. Prescribing in Pregnancy, fourth ed. BMJ Books/Blackwell Publishing, Oxford.

Schaefer, C., Peters, P.W.J., Miller, R.K. (Eds.), 2007. Drugs during Pregnancy and Lactation: Treatment Options and Risk Assessment, Academic Press/Elsevier, London.

SPC from the eMC, Buscopan® tablets, Boehringer Ingelheim Ltd, updated on the eMC 14/2/12.

SPC from the eMC, Co-Codamol BP Tablets, Wockhardt UK Ltd, updated on eMC 26/3/12.

SPC from the eMC, Codeine Phosphate 15 mg, 30 mg and 60 mg tablets, Actavis UK Ltd, updated on the eMC 23/2/11.

SPC from the eMC, Co-Dydramol Tablets, Actavis UK Ltd, updated on the eMC 7/10/11.

SPC from the eMC, Diamorphine Hydrochloride injection, Auralis Ltd, updated on the eMC 15/2/10.

SPC from the eMC, Diclofenac Sodium BP tablets 75 mg (SR) and 100 mg (Retard), Novartis Pharmaceuticals UK Ltd, updated on the eMC 26/7/11.

SPC from the eMC, Dihydrocodeine 30 mg tablets, Goldshield Group UK Ltd, updated on the eMC 18/8/10.

SPC from the eMC, Distalgesic® tablets, Dista Products Ltd, updated on the eMC 13/08/01.

SPC from the eMC, Fentanyl Injection 50 mcg/mL, Goldshield Group Ltd, updated on the eMC17/1/11.

SPC from the eMC, Ibuprofen 400 mg and 600 mg, Abbott Healthcare Products Ltd, updated on the eMC 24/1/11.

SPC from the eMC, Meptid injection 100 mg/mL, Almirall Ltd, updated on the eMC 9/5/11.

SPC from the eMC, Morphine Sulphate Injection BP 10 mg/mL; 15 mg/mL; 30 mg/mL, Wockhardt UK Ltd, updated on the eMC 9/4/10.

SPC from the eMC, Oramorph oral solution 10 mg/5 mL Boehringer Ingelheim Ltd, updated on the eMC 22/9/12.

SPC from the eMC, Paracetamol 500 mg Tablets, Actavis UK Ltd, updated on the eMC 2/2/11.

SPC from the eMC, Paracetamol Oral suspension 120 mg in 5 mL, Pinewood Healthcare, updated on eMC 19/4/11.

SPC from the eMC Pethidine Hydrochloride Injection 100 mg in 2 mL, Goldshield Group Ltd, updated on the eMC 13/7/09.

SPC from the eMC, Ponstan™ Tablets 250 or 500 mg, Chemidex Pharma Ltd, updated on the eMC 12/3/10.

SPC from the eMC, Soluble Aspirin BP Tablets 300 mg, Actavis UK Ltd, updated on eMC 1/3/11.

Volans, G., Wiseman, H., 2012. Drugs Handbook 2012–2013, thirty-third ed. Palgrave Macmillan, Basingstoke.

Further Reading

Bartholomew, C., Yerby, M., 2011. Pain, Labour and Women's Choice of Pain Relief. In: Macdonald, S., Magill-Cuerden, J. (Eds.), Mayes' Midwifery, fourteenth ed. Baillière Tindall/Elsevier, Edinburgh, pp. 521–534.

Yerby, M., 2000. Pain Management in Childbearing: Key Issues in Management. Baillière Tindall/Elsevier, Edinburgh.

3

Antacids

These drugs/preparations are used to reduce gastric acidity and give relief from heartburn when changes in diet and posture have no effect. They may also be used as prophylaxis prior to the induction of anaesthesia where there is a risk of Mendelson syndrome, i.e. before either elective or emergency caesarean section.

Antacids should not be taken at the same time as other medication as they impair absorption.

H_2 antagonists act upon histamine receptors and can intensify or aggravate an asthmatic response. They should be used with caution in hepatic and or renal impairment.

The student should be aware of:

- the effect of progesterone on the mother
- local protocols for management of high-risk clients during labour
- the procedure of applying 'cricoid pressure' during induction of anaesthesia
- updated resuscitation techniques
- the effects of narcotic analgesia on gastric emptying.

BP
Cimetidine

Proprietary
Dyspamet® (Goldshield Pharmaceuticals Ltd), Tagamet® (SmithKline Beecham), cimetidine (non-proprietary, see BNF for details)

Continued

Group
Antacid, H$_2$ receptor antagonist

Uses/indications
To reduce gastric acidity, intrapartum or prior to caesarean section

Type of drug
POM

Presentation
Tablets – light green, also chewable and effervescent, IM injection, syrup

Dosage
Oral – 400 mg at start of labour repeated 4 hrly (max 2.4 g/day)
IM – 200 mg 4–6-hrly (max dosage 2.4 g daily), IV – slow injection 200 mg over at least 5 min 4–6-hrly, IV infusion – 50–100 mg/h over 24 h

Route of admin
Oral, IM, rarely IV slow injection or IV infusion

Contraindications
Hypersensitivity to cimetidine, avoid in clients stabilized on phenytoin and warfarin

Side effects
Rare but include dizziness, rash, in high doses reversible confusional states, headache

Interactions
Analgesics – inhibits the metabolism of opioid analgesics and increases their plasma concentration
Antibiotics – inhibits the metabolism of metronidazole and erythromycin
Anticoagulants – inhibits the metabolism of warfarin, and enhances its effects
Antiepileptics – inhibits the metabolism of phenytoin, sodium valproate and carbamazepine
Antihypertensives – inhibits the metabolism of labetalol

Pharmacodynamic properties
H_2 receptor antagonist that rapidly inhibits both basal and stimulated gastric secretion of acid. It also reduces pepsin output

Fetal risk
No evidence to suggest cimetidine is hazardous but it should be avoided unless necessary

Breastfeeding

Excreted in breast milk but not known to be harmful

BP
Ranitidine

Proprietary
Zantac® (GlaxoSmithKlein UK), contains sodium

Group
Antacid, H_2 antagonist

Uses/indications
reduces gastric acidity in high-risk labours, prior to caesarean section or any other surgical procedure. Prophylaxis of acid aspiration (Mendelson's) syndrome: 150 mg oral dose can be given 2 h before anaesthesia, and preferably also 150 mg the previous evening. Alternatively, the injection is also available.
In obstetric patients in labour 150 mg every 6 h, but if general anaesthesia is required it is recommended that a non-particulate antacid (e.g. sodium citrate) be given in addition. The usual precautions to avoid acid aspiration should also be taken.

Type of drug
POM

Presentation
Tablets (also dispersible or effervescent), syrup, injection

Continued

Dosage
150 mg at onset of labour, repeat 6 hrly or see protocols, IM or slow IV 50 mg 45–60 min prior to the induction of analgesia, IV injection 20 mL over 2 min

Route of admin
Oral, IM, IV injection

Contraindications
As for cimetidine, hypersensitivity

Side effects
As for cimetidine, rarely tachycardia, and with long-term use agitation and visual disturbances

Interactions
As for cimetidine, but effects less likely

Pharmacodynamic properties
As for cimetidine, relatively long-acting. Ranitidine is a specific, rapidly acting, histamine H_2 antagonist. It inhibits basal and stimulated secretion of gastric acid, reducing both the volume and the acid and pepsin content of the secretion. Ranitidine has a relatively long duration of action and so a single 150 mg dose effectively suppresses gastric acid secretion for 12 h.

Fetal risk
Crosses the placenta and should only be used in the long term only if essential, for prophylaxis in labour or LSCS. No adverse effect has been reported on labour, delivery or neonatal period

Breastfeeding
Excreted in significant amounts but not known to be harmful

BP
Alginic acid

Proprietary
Gaviscon® Advance (Forum Health Products Ltd) –
aniseed flavour

Group
Antacid – alginate

Uses/indications
Dyspepsia, cardiac reflux (heartburn)

Type of drug
GSL

Presentation
Tablets, oral suspension – peppermint, or aniseed

Dosage
Tablets 1–2 as required, or 10–20 mL as required

Route of admin
Oral

Contraindications
Hypersensitivity

Side effects
No data available, but caution in a sodium-restricted
diet

Interactions
Impaired absorption of oral iron

Pharmacodynamic properties
Alginic acid reacts with the gastric acid to form a
pH-neutral gel raft over the stomach contents and is
effective for up to 4 h

Fetal risk
Nil known from research studies, although manufacturer recommends limit treatment as much as possible

Breastfeeding
Not secreted in breast milk

References and Recommended Reading

Baxter, K., 2011. Stockley's Drug Interaction Companion. Pharmaceutical Press, London.

Briggs, G., Freeman, R., Yaffe, S., 2008. Drugs in pregnancy and lactation: a reference guide to fetal and neonatal risk, eighth ed. Lippincott Williams and Wilkins, Philadelphia.

Bubimschi, C., Weiner, C., 2010. Medication. In: James, D.K., Steer, P.J., Weiner, C.P., Gonik, B. (Eds.), High Risk Pregnancy: Management Options, fourth ed. Elsevier Saunders, London, pp. 579–598.

Hofmeyr, G.J., Neilson, J.P., Alfreirevic, Z., Crowther, C., Duley, L., Gulmezoglu, M., Gyte, G.M., Hodnett, E.D. 2008. Pregnancy and Childbirth – a Cochrane Pocketbook. Wiley Cochrane Series, London.

Joint Formulary Committee, 2011. British National Formulary (BNF) 62. Pharmaceutical Press, London.

Jordan, S., 2010. Management of gastric acidity in pregnancy. In: Jordan, S. (Ed.), Pharmacology for Midwives: The Evidence Base for Safe Practice, second ed. Palgrave Macmillan, Basingstoke, pp. 263–270.

Koren, G., 2007. Medication Safety in Pregnancy and Breastfeeding: The Evidence Based A–Z Clinician's Pocket Guide. McGraw-Hill, New York.

Rubin, P.C., Ramsey, M., 2007. Prescribing in Pregnancy, fourth ed. BMJ Books/Blackwell Publishing, Oxford.

Schaefer, C., Peters, P.W.J., Miller, R.K. (Eds.), 2007. Drugs During Pregnancy and Lactation: Treatment Options and Risk Assessment, Academic Press/Elsevier, London.

SPC from the eMC, Liquid Gaviscon®; Liquid Gaviscon® – peppermint flavour, Gaviscon Advance, Britannia Pharmaceuticals Ltd, updated on the eMC 13/8/10.

SPC from the eMC, Tagamet® 400 mg and 800 mg tablets, 400 mg effervescent tablets, syrup, injection, Chemidex Pharma Ltd, updated on the eMC 18/3/09.

SPC from the eMC, Zantac® tablets 150 mg, GlaxoSmithKlein UK, updated on the eMC 16/12/10.

Vamer, R.G., 1993. Mechanisms of regurgitation and its prevention with cricoid pressure. International Journal of Obstetrical Anaesthesia 2, 207–215.

Volans, G., Wiseman, H., 2012. Drugs Handbook 2012–2013, thirtythird ed. Palgrave Macmillan, Basingstoke.

Further Reading

Centre for Maternal and Child Enquiries 2011 Saving Mothers' Lives, Reviewing maternal deaths to make motherhood safer: 2006–2008. The 8th Report of the Confidential Enquiries into Maternal Deaths in the United Kingdom. Available http://www.oaa-anaes.ac.uk/assets/_managed/editor/File/Reports/2006-2008%20CEMD.pdf [accessed 2 March 2012]

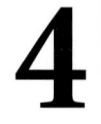

4

Antibiotics

Antibiotics are produced by certain bacteria or fungi that interfere with or prevent the growth of other bacteria/fungi. They are used in infection or as prophylaxis, e.g. in cases of spontaneous rupture of membranes longer than 24 hours, or in lower-segment caesarean section.

The student should be aware of:

- causes and transmission of infection
- causal organisms of infection and their laboratory identification
- the symptoms and progression of infection
- the importance of bacterial culture and sensitivity
- the ingestion, uptake, action and excretion of the prescribed drug
- the NICE guideline on prophylaxis for infective endocarditis (CG 064) (2008), which recommended that antibiotics should not be given for dental or other interventional procedures, e.g. obstetric/gynaecological procedure(s) or childbirth
- group B streptococcal guidance
- preterm prelabour rupture of membranes guidance.

BP
Metronidazole

Proprietary
Flagyl® (Winthrop Pharmaceuticals UK Ltd) (Aventis UK Ltd), Metrolyl® (Sandoz Ltd), Flagyl® injection (Winthrop Pharmaceuticals UK Ltd), metronidazole (non-proprietary, see BNF for details)

Group
Antimicrobial

Uses/indications
Treatment of anaerobic infection with a wide range of activity, prophylaxis in surgery (anaerobic bacteria and anaerobic streptococci), clostridium, *Trichomonas vaginalis, Eubacterium, Gardnerella vaginalis,* puerperal sepsis, bacterial vaginosis, gingivitis

Type of drug
POM

Presentation
Tablets, suspension, suppositories, pre-prepared IV injections and infusions

Dosage
Oral: stat 800 mg then 400–500 mg t.d.s.
IV: 500 mg t.d.s.
P.R.: 1 g t.d.s. for 3 days max, then 1 g b.d. treatment of bacterial vaginosis as for oral, or 2 g single dose

Route of admin
Oral, P.R., IV, IM

Contraindications
In pregnancy and breastfeeding avoid high dosage, avoid alcohol, known hypersensitivity to metronidazole

Side effects
Unpleasant taste in mouth, furry tongue, nausea, vomiting, rashes, headache, drowsiness, dizziness, dark urine and, very rarely, angio-oedema

Interactions
Alcohol – disulfiram-like reaction – avoid during treatment and for 48 h post course
Antacids – cimetidine inhibits the metabolism of metronidazole
Anticoagulants – enhances the effect of warfarin but no interaction with heparin
Antiepileptics – inhibits the metabolism of phenytoin; phenobarbital accelerates metabolism of metronidazole

Oestrogens – reduces the effect of the combined oral contraceptive pill

Pharmacodynamic properties
Antimicrobial effective against a wide range of infections with antiprotozoal and antibacterial actions

Fetal risk
Avoid high-dose regimens; use in first trimester can cause midline facial defects, cardiac defects, genital defects and limb defects, but has been used with little effect in last two trimesters

Breastfeeding
Significant amounts secreted; avoid large single doses

BP
Erythromycin stearate

Proprietary
Erythrocin® (Amdipharm PLC)
Erythromycin (non-proprietary, see BNF for details)

Group
Antibiotic, macrolide

Uses/indications
Used in penicillin-sensitive clients, penicillin-resistant organisms, syphilis, chlamydia, gonorrhoea, respiratory infection, treatment of infection sensitive to erythromycin, prophylaxis in management of pre-term rupture of membranes

Type of drug
POM

Presentation
Tablets, capsules, powder for reconstitution, granules, suspension

Dosage
1–2 g/day in even doses, depending on the severity of infection
Oral: 250–500 mg q.d.s. or 0.5–1 g b.d.

Syphilis/chlamydia: 500 mg q.d.s. for 14 days; IV:
25–50 mg/kg daily or 1–2 g in 6 even doses

Route of admin
Oral, IV

Contraindications
Hypersensitivity, hepatic dysfunction

Side effects
Nausea, vomiting, diarrhoea, fever, skin eruptions,
urticaria, rashes, cardiac arrhythmias; in large doses –
reversible hearing loss, hepatic dysfunction, thrombophlebitis following IV administration, allergic response
rare with mild anaphylaxis

Interactions
Anticoagulants – effect of warfarin enhanced
Antihistamines – inhibits the metabolism of terfenadine,
causing dangerous cardiac arrhythmias
Cisapride – can cause cardiotoxicity and arrhythmias
Ergotamines – acute ergot toxicity, rapid peripheral
vasospasm and dysaesthesia
Theophylline – inhibition of metabolism of theophylline

Pharmacodynamic properties
Antimicrobial that attaches to a subunit of susceptible
organisms and suppresses protein synthesis, destroying cell
wall stability and making them vulnerable to attack. Active
against both Gram-positive and Gram-negative bacteria,
mycoplasms, treponema, chlamydia and gonorrhoea

Fetal risk
Crosses the placental barrier but not in appreciable
quantities; fetal concentrations have found to be low,
with no reports of congenital defects located except in
animal studies – cardiovascular malformations if used in
early pregnancy. However, manufacturers advise that, if
used to treat maternal syphilitic infection during
pregnancy, the infant may be born with congenital
syphilis and should receive penicillin treatment
following birth

Breastfeeding
Secreted in only small amounts in breast milk
– considered safe with no ill effects reported, although
manufacturers advise avoidance

BP
Cefuroxime

Proprietary
Cefuroxime (Sandoz Ltd); Zinacef (GlaxoSmithKlein
UK),
Cephradine (non-proprietary, see BNF for details)

Group
Antibiotic – cephalosporin

Uses/indications
Against both Gram-positive and Gram-negative
bacteria, prophylaxis with LSCS, UTI, respiratory
infections

Type of drug
POM

Presentation
Capsules, syrup, powder for reconstitution

Dosage
Oral: 250–500 mg b.d. or 0.5–1 g b.d.
IM, IV: 500 mg–1 g q.d.s. given over 3–5 min

Route of admin
Oral, IM, IV

Contraindications
Renal dysfunction, known hypersensitivity to cephalosporins, caution in penicillin hypersensitivity

Side effects
Nausea, diarrhoea and hypersensitivity – usually mild,
headache, dizziness, dyspnoea

Interactions
Nil specific to cephradine:

Anticoagulants – effect of warfarin enhanced

Uricosurics – excretion is reduced by probenecid

Oestrogens – reduces the effect of the combined oral contraceptive pill

Pharmacodynamic properties
Broad-spectrum bactericidal drug active against Gram-positive organisms, e.g. staphylococci, streptococci, *Streptococcus pyogenes, Streptococcus pneumoniae,* and Gram-negative organisms such as *Escherichia coli, Haemophilus influenzae,* salmonella. Highly active against penicillinase-producing staphylococci. e.g. *S. aureus*

Fetal risk
No reports of congenital defects located, although manufacturers advise safety not established

Breastfeeding
Considered safe, although manufacturers advise caution – as for amoxicillin

---

BP
Flucloxacillin sodium

Proprietary
Floxapen® (Actavis UK Ltd), flucloxacillin (Aurobinda Pharma Ltd) (non-proprietary, see BNF for details)

Group
Antibiotic, penicillinase-resistant penicillin

Uses/indications
Against β-lactamase Gram-positive resistant microbes, including *S. aureus* and streptococci; prophylaxis in surgery

Type of drug
POM

Presentation
Capsules, syrup, powder for reconstitution

Continued

Dosage
Oral: 250–500 mg t.d.s. (30–60 min before food)
IV/infusion: 250 mg–2 g q.d.s.
IM: 250–500 mg q.d.s. (according to severity of infection)
Prophylaxis: 1–2 g IV at induction of anaesthesia, then
500 mg q.d.s. IM or IV for up to 72 h

Route of admin
Oral, IM, IV/infusion

Contraindications
Penicillin and/or cephalosporin hypersensitivity,
sodium-restricted diet, renal or hepatic impairment

Side effects
Anaphylaxis – uncommon and usually mild and
transitory, diarrhoea, rash, indigestion, rarely hepatic
impairment, reversible neutropenia, thrombocytopenia

Interactions
Contraceptives – reduces contraceptive effect

Pharmacodynamic properties
Narrow-spectrum penicillin that is not inactivated by
staphylococcal lactamases. It acts on the synthesis of the
bacterial wall and exerts a bactericidal effect on streptococci, including *Neisseria* and *Clostridia,* but not MRSA

Fetal risk
Animal studies show no teratogenicity but manufacturer advises that it should be withheld unless
considered essential

Breastfeeding
Trace quantities can be detected in breast milk;
considered safe, but as for amoxicillin

BP
Co-amoxiclav (compound of Amoxicillin as a sodium
salt and Clavulanic acid)

Proprietary
Augmentin® (GlaxoSmithKline UK)

Group
Antibiotic, broad-spectrum penicillinase

Uses/indications
Against bacteria resistant to amoxicillin, i.e.
S. aureus, E. coli, gonorrhoea, β-lactamase infection, UTI,
abdominal infection, cellulitis, prophylaxis at LSCS or MRP

Type of drug
POM

Presentation
Tablets, dispersible tablets, suspension, powder for
reconstitution

Dosage
Oral: 375 mg (250 mg expressed as amoxicillin) t.d.s.;
625 mg (500 mg) t.d.s in severe infection
IV: 600 mg–1.2 g t.d.s.

Route of admin
Oral, IV, IV infusion

Contraindications
Penicillin and/or cephalosporin hypersensitivity,
jaundice/hepatic dysfunction

Side effects
Nausea, diarrhoea, rashes, rarely hepatic impairment,
hypersensitivity, CNS effects – rare, vaginal itching,
soreness and discharge

Interactions
Nil specific
Anticoagulants – may prolong bleeding time and
prothrombin time
Contraceptives – reduces contraceptive effect

Pharmacodynamic properties
Resistance to antibiotics is caused by bacterial enzymes
destroying it before it is able to act on the pathogen.
The clavulanate anticipates this and blocks β-lactamase
enzymes in organisms sensitive to amoxicillin.
Co-amoxiclav has a rapid bactericidal effect

Continued

Fetal risk
Animal studies with oral and parenteral administration
show no teratogenicity, but manufacturers advise
avoidance in the first trimester and use thereafter only
when considered essential; second/third trimesters – a
single study of women with preterm premature rupture
of membranes given Augmentin for prophylaxis against
infection found an association with necrotizing
enterocolitis in the neonate (SPC – Augmentin® 8/6/10)

Breastfeeding
Little known of effects of clavulanic acid on breastfed
infants; trace quantities of amoxicillin excreted but
considered safe – as for amoxicillin

BP
Amoxicillin trihydrate

Proprietary
Amoxil® (GlaxoSmithKline UK)

Group
Antibiotic, broad-spectrum penicillinase

Uses/indications
Broad spectrum; used against aerobes Gram-positive
(e.g. *Streptococcus*, *Staphylococcus* and *Listerisa
monocytogenes*) and Gram-negative bacteria (e.g.
Haemophilus influenza, *E.schericha coli* and *Salmonella*
species, except *Pseudomonas*), and anaerobes (e.g.
Closteridium); also respiratory infections, UTI, gonorrhoea,
puerperal sepsis

Type of drug
POM

Presentation
Capsules, dispersible tablets, suspension – paediatric
and adult, powder for reconstitution

Dosage
Oral: 250–500 mg t.d.s.
IM: 500 mg t.d.s.

IV: 500 mg t.d.s. to 1 g q.d.s. in severe infection
Prophylaxis with heart valves, etc.: 1 g IV, then 500 mg
6 hrs later

Route of admin
Oral, IM, IV/infusion

Contraindications
Penicillin hypersensitivity

Side effects
Mild diarrhoea, indigestion, rash, rarely anaphylaxis
– usually mild

Interactions
Anticoagulants – causes prolonged prothrombin time
Contraceptives – reduces contraceptive effect
Uricosurics – excretion reduced with concomitant
administration of probenecid, – used in treatment of
gonorrhoea

Pharmacodynamic properties
Broad spectrum antibiotic with rapid bactericidal
effects; which has the safety profile of penicillin

Fetal risk
Nil known, no reports of toxicity in animal or human
studies, but manutacturers advise benefits should
outweigh the risks

Breastfeeding
Considered safe but modifies the bowel flora and can
cause sensitizaton; interferes with culture results if an
infection screen is required

BP
Trimethoprim

Proprietary
Co-trimoxazole® (Actavis UK Ltd)
Trimethoprim (non-proprietary, see BNF for details)

Group
Antimicrobial – sulphonamide

Uses/indications
Treatment of sensitive organisms, UTI, URTI, prophylaxis against UTI

Type of drug
POM

Presentation
Tablets, suspension, injection

Dosage
Oral: 100–200 mg b.d.
IV injection/infusion: 200 mg b.d.
Prophylaxis: 200 mg

Route of admin
Oral, IV

Contraindications
Pregnancy, hypersensitivity to trimethoprim, blood dyscrasias, renal insufficiency or impairment

Side effects
Nausea, vomiting, rash – mild and reversible, allergic reactions, including anaphylaxis

Interactions
Anticonvulsants – half-life of phenytoin is increased, antifolate effect enhanced
Anticoagulants – enhanced anticoagulant effect
Oestrogens – reduces the effect of the combined oral contraceptive pill

Pharmacodynamic properties
Antimicrobial that which works by selective inhibition of bacterial dihydrofolate reductase. It is effective against both Gram-positive and Gram-negative aerobic organisms, including *E. coli, Proteus, Klebsiella, S. aureus, Streptococcus. faecalis* and *pneumoniae, Haemophilus influenzae*, but NOT *Neisseria, Pseudomonas aeruginosa, Treponema pallidum* or anaerobes

Fetal risk
First trimester: teratogen – as a folate antagonist, manufacturers advise avoidance as can cause transient hyperbilirubinaemia in the neonate (Bubimschi & and Weiner, 2010)

Breastfeeding
Excreted in small amounts but considered moderately safe in the short term

---

BP
Gentamicin sulphate

Proprietary
Gentamicin (Hospira UK Ltd); Cidomycin® (Sanofi-Aventis); Genticin injectable (Amdipharm PLC)

Group
Broad-spectrum aminoglycoside antibiotic

Uses/indications
Gram-positive and Gram-negative pathogens, systemic infection, prophylaxis during labour for patients with heart valves/heart disease, UTI, chest infection

Type of drug
POM

Presentation
Ampoules

Dosage
3–4 mg/kg body weight daily in divided doses (e.g. 80 mg 8-hrly in patients over 60 kg, or 60 mg 8-hrly in those under 60 kg)

Route of admin
IM, IV slow injection, IV infusion

Contraindications
Hypersensitivity, myasthenia gravis, renal impairment

Side effects
Toxicity – renal toxicity reversible after withdrawal. Vestibular hearing loss/damage, hypersensitivity

Interactions
Avoid concomitant use with ototoxic and nephrotoxic drugs

Muscle relaxants – enhances the muscle relaxant effect

Oestrogens – may reduce the effect of the combined oral contraceptive pill

Pharmacodynamic properties
Bactericidal aminoglycoside that acts by inhibiting protein synthesis, acting on the integrity of the plasma membrane and metabolism of ribonucleic acid

Fetal risk
Safety is not established and it crosses the placental barrier second/third trimester – probably low risk but potentially may cause deafness

Breastfeeding
Present in breast milk, and although unlikely to cause problems the manufacturers advise avoidance

---

BP
Benzylpenicillin

Proprietary
(Penicillin G) Crystapen® (Genus Pharmaceuticals)

Group
Antibiotic – penicillinase

Uses/indications
Streptococcal infection, i.e. throat infection, ear infection, pneumonia, treatment of gonorrhoea

Type of drug
POM

Presentation
Vials of powder for reconstitution

Dosage
IM, IV injection or IV infusion: 2.4–4.8 g in four divided doses (available in 600 mg and 1200 mg doses equivalent to 1 and 2 megaunits)

Route of admin
IM, IV injection/infusion

Contraindications
Hypersensitivity to penicillin

Side effects
Hypersensitivity – urticaria, fever, joint pain, rashes, anaphylaxis, diarrhoea, thrombocytopenia, neutropenia, haemolytic anaemia – in high doses

Interactions
Nil specific
Oestrogens – reduces the effect of combined oral contraceptive pill

Pharmacodynamic properties
Bacteriostatic with bactericidal activities against Gram-negative coli. It is inactivated by gastric acid and is therefore best given IV or by injection

Fetal risk
Nil reported

Breastfeeding
No data available from controlled studies in breastfeeding women, although it is considered safe

---

BP
Ampicillin

Proprietary
Penbritin® (Chemidex Pharma Ltd)
Ampicillin (non-proprietary, see BNF for details)

Group
Broad-spectrum antibiotic, penicillin

Uses/indications
Wide range of bacterial infections including UTI, ear infection, sinusitis, bronchitis, *Haemophilus influenzae,* salmonella, meningococcal disease, listerial meningitis

Type of drug
POM

Presentation
Capsules, suspension, vials for injection

Dosage
Oral: 0.25–1 g q.d.s. (taken 30 min before food)
IM, IV/IVI: 500 mg 4–6-hrly

Route of admin
Oral, IM, IV

Contraindications
Hypersensitivity to penicillin, history of renal impairment, caution with erythematous rash

Side effects
Gastrointestinal disturbances, rashes, hypersensitivity – anaphylaxis

Interactions
Antibiotics – concurrent use of bacteriostatic drugs can interfere with the bactericidal action of ampicillin
Anticoagulants – INR may be altered by course of broad-spectrum antibiotics
Oestrogens – reduces the effectiveness of combined oral contraceptive pill

Pharmacodynamic properties
Broad-spectrum antibiotic indicated in the treatment of a wide range of bacterial infections caused by ampicillin-sensitive organisms

Fetal risk
Manufacturer advises documentary evidence of clinical use in pregnancy extensively since 1961 with no shown teratogenic effects

Breastfeeding
Trace amounts excreted into breast milk, but there are no adequate data about use during lactation; no advice regarding avoidance

References and Recommended Reading

Baxter, K., 2011. Stockley's Drug Interaction Companion. Pharmaceutical Press, London.

Briggs, G., Freeman, R., Yaffe, S., 2008. Drugs in Pregnancy and Lactation: A Reference Guide to Fetal and Neonatal Risk, eighth ed. Lippincott Williams and Wilkins, Philadelphia.

Bubimschi, C., Weiner, C., 2010. Medication. In: James, D.K., Steer, P.J., Weiner, C.P., Gonik, B. (Eds.), High Risk Pregnancy: Management Options, fourth ed. Elsevier Saunders, London, pp. 579–598.

Joint Formulary Committee, 2011. British National Formulary (BNF) 62. Pharmaceutical Press, London.

Koren, G., 2007. Medication Safety in Pregnancy and Breastfeeding: The Evidence Based A–Z Clinician's Pocket Guide. McGraw-Hill, New York.

National Institute for Health and Clinical Excellence (NICE), 2007. CG 55 Intrapartum Care. NICE, London.

National Institute for Health and Clinical Excellence (NICE), 2007. CG 70 Induction of Labour. NICE, London.

Royal College of Obstetricians and Gynaecologists (RCOG), 2003. Prevention of Early Onset Neonatal Group B Streptococcal Disease. Greentop Guideline No. 36. RCOG, London.

Royal College of Obstetricians and Gynaecologists (RCOG), 2006. Preterm Pre-labour Rupture of Membranes. Greentop Guideline No. 44. RCOG, London.

Rubin, P.C., Ramsey, M., 2007. Prescribing in Pregnancy, fourth ed. BMJ Books/Blackwell Publishing, Oxford.

Schaefer, C., Peters, P.W.J., Miller, R.K., 2007. Drugs During Pregnancy and Lactation: Treatment Options and Risk Assessment. Academic Press/Elsevier, London.

SPC from the eMC, Amoxil®, Glaxo 250 mg and 500 mg capsules GlaxoSmithKline UK, updated on the eMC 23/11/10.

SPC from the eMC, Augmentin® IV, 375 mg or 625 mg tablets and suspension, GlaxoSmithKline UK, updated on the eMC 8/6/10.

SPC from the eMC, Cefuroxime®, 250 mg tablets, Sandoz Ltd, updated on the eMC 28/9/10.

SPC from the eMC, Co-trimoxazole 80 mg with Sulfamethoxazole 400 mg tablets, Actavis UK Ltd, updated on the eMC 30/11/10.

SPC from the eMC, Crystapen®, injection 600 mg and 1200 mg vials, Genus Pharmaceuticals, updated on the eMC 16/9/08.

SPC from the eMC, Erythrocin®, 250 mg tablets, Amdipharm PLC, updated on the eMC 10/11/10.

SPC from the eMC, Flagyl®, 200 mg and 400 mg tablets and suspension, Winthrop Pharmaceuticals UK Ltd, updated on the eMC 17/5/11.

SPC from the eMC, Flagyl® 500 mg and 1 g suppositories, Winthrop Pharmaceuticals UK Ltd, updated on the eMC 17/5/11.

SPC from the eMC, Flagyl® injection 500 mg/100 mL, Winthrop Pharmaceuticals UK Ltd, updated on the eMC 17/5/11.

SPC from the eMC, Floxapen® capsules, syrup, vials for injection, Actavis UK Ltd, updated on the eMC 25/1/10.

SPC from the eMC, Flucloxacillin 125/5 mL solution, 250 mg and 500 mg capsules, Aurobinda Pharma Ltd, updated on the eMC 24/8/11.

SPC from the eMC, Gentamycin® 40 mg/mL injection, Hospira UK Ltd, updated on the eMC 22/8/11.

SPC from the eMC, Penbritin® vials 500 mg, capsules 250 mg and 500 mg, Chemiddex Pharma Ltd, updated on the eMC 4/2/09.

SPC from the eMC, Trimethoprim® 100 mg and 200 mg tablets, Accord Healthcare Ltd, updated on the eMC 9/2/12.

SPC from the eMC, Zinacef® 250 mg, 750 mg, 1.5 g injection, GlaxoSmithKlein UK, updated on the eMC 19/11/08.

Tomlinson, M.W., 2010. Cardiac disease. In: James, D.K., Steer, P.J., Weiner, C.P., Gonik, B. (Eds.), High Risk Pregnancy: Management Options, fourth ed. Elsevier Saunders, London, pp. 627–656.

Tutt, M., Jordan, S., 2010. Antimicrobial agents. In: Jordan, S. (Ed.), Pharmacology for Midwives: The Evidence Base for Safe Practice, second ed. Palgrave Macmillan, Basingstoke, pp. 284–307.

Volans, G., Wiseman, H., 2012. Drugs Handbook 2012–2013, thirtythird ed. Palgrave Macmillan, Basingstoke.

Yudin, M., 2010. Other infectious conditions in pregnancy. In: James, D.K., Steer, P.J., Weiner, C.P., Gonik, B. (Eds.), High Risk Pregnancy: Management Options, fourth ed. Elsevier Saunders, London, pp. 521–542.

Further Reading

Centre for Maternal and Child Enquiries, 2011. Saving Mothers' Lives: Reviewing Maternal Deaths to Make Motherhood Safer: 2006–2008. The 8th Report of the Confidential Enquiries into Maternal Deaths in the United Kingdom. Available http://www.oaa-anaes.ac.uk/assets/_managed/editor/File/Reports/2006-2008%20CEMD.pdf [accessed 2 March 2012].

5

Anticoagulants

Anticoagulants are substances used to prevent blood clotting.
The student should be aware of:

- factors predisposing to thromboembolism
- local protocols for management of thromboembolism
- the antagonist for such treatment and its availability
- factors involved in the mechanism of blood clotting, and the criteria used to determine which is the most appropriate anticoagulant
- conditions requiring treatment with anticoagulants
- maternal and fetal sequelae of such treatment
- the effects of progesterone on the circulatory system.

Heparin antagonist: protamine sulphate
Warfarin antagonist: vitamin K and plasma

BP Heparin (as sodium or calcium salt)
Proprietary Heparin Sodium (Wockhardt UK Ltd)
Group Anticoagulant, parenteral
Uses/indications Treatment of DVT, pulmonary embolism, thromboembolism – susceptible clients, prophylaxis in LSCS or high risk due to impaired mobility
Type of drug POM

Continued

Presentation
Preloaded syringes, vials or ampoules

Dosage
IV: 5000 units loading dose and then continuous infusion of 15–25 units/kg/hr adjusted by laboratory monitoring (severe PE: loading dose 10 000 units)
S.C.: after LSCS 5000 units b.d. until ambulant during pregnancy: 5–10 000 units b.d. – monitoring required
DVT: 15 000 units b.d.

Route of admin
S.C., IV

Contraindications
Haemorrhagic disorders, including heparin-induced thrombocytopenia, cerebral aneurysm, cerebral vascular accident/cerebral haemorrhage, severe hypertension, peptic ulcer, haemophilia, liver disease, major trauma, hypersensitivity, threatened abortion

Side effects
Haemorrhage, including placental sites, thrombocytopenia hypersensitivity, bruising and haematoma formation. Prolonged use is associated with osteoporosis

Interactions
Nil specific
Anticoagulants – concomitant use enhances effects: use caution when transferring to oral anticoagulants
Antihistamines – decreases the anticoagulant effect
Aspirin – antiplatelet effect enhanced by heparin
Diclofenac – increased risk of haemorrhage (with IV diclofenac)
GTN – the excretion of heparin is increased by the GTN decreasing the anticoagulant effect
NSAIDs IV – possible increased risk of bleeding

Pharmacodynamic properties

A naturally occurring anticoagulant that is synthesized and excreted by mast cells in the body. It acts by forming a complex with antithrombin, catalysing the inhibition of several activated blood coagulation factors and thrombin. This prevents the conversion of fibrinogen to fibrin, which is crucial for clot formation. The onset of action is immediate; and it is most commonly used for the prevention and treatment of venous and arterial thromboembolism

Fetal risk

Available data suggest there is no risk to fetus or neonate

Breastfeeding

Not excreted in breast milk

NB: discontinue use prior to peridural anaesthesia, i.e. 8–12 h; can cause spinal haematoma or permanent paralysis

OVERDOSE

Indicated by haemorrhage; APTT and platelet count should be determined. Minor haemorrhage rarely requires specific treatment; and decreasing or delaying subsequent doses of heparin should be sufficient. Major haemorrhage: the anticoagulant effect is reduced immediately by 1% protamine sulphate, but caution is required as protamine also has an anticoagulant effect. A single dose should never exceed 50 mg

IV injection of protamine can cause a sudden fall in blood pressure, bradycardia, dyspnoea and transitory flushing, but this can be avoided or decreased by slow and careful administration

BP
Warfarin sodium

Proprietary
Marevan® (Goldshield Group Ltd),
Warfarin sodium (non-proprietary, see BNF for details)

Group
Anticoagulant – oral

Uses/indications
Prophylaxis after prosthetic heart valve surgery, DVT,
pulmonary embolism, and transient ischaemic attacks

Type of drug
POM

Presentation
Tablets, white 0.5 mg, brown 1 mg, blue 3 mg, pink
5 mg

Dosage
Refer to pharmacist or BNF; usually 3–10 mg daily

Route of admin
Oral

Contraindications
Pregnancy, but may be used between 16 and 36 weeks'
gestation if heparin not available and risks of thrombosis outweigh the risk to the fetus; peptic ulcer, severe
hypertension, bacterial endocarditis, haemorrhage; use
within 24 h of surgery or labour – caution if needed

Side effects
Haemorrhage, nausea, transient alopecia, hypersensitivity, fall in haematocrit, purple toes, liver dysfunction,
pancreatitis

Interactions

Alcohol – enhanced effects with large alcohol doses

Antacids – cimetidine inhibits the metabolism and enhances the effect of warfarin

Aspirin – increased risk of haemorrhage – antiplatelet effect

Antibiotics – cephalosporins, macrolides, erythromycin and metronidazole, sulphonamides, trimethoprim – possible enhanced coagulant effect

Penicillins – possible alteration of INR

Antidepressants – SSRIs – anticoagulant effect increased

Dextropropoxyphene – anticoagulant effect enhanced

Paracetamol – theoretical increased risk of bleeds with prolonged use

Cholestyramine – enhanced anticoagulant effect

Barbiturates – metabolism of warfarin increased, therefore diminishes the anticoagulant effect

Antiepileptics – carbamazepine and phenobarbital – diminishes the anticoagulant effect

Phenytoin – both enhances and diminishes warfarin's effect

Sodium valproate – enhanced anticoagulant effect

Oral contraceptive – diminished contraceptive effect

NSAIDs – enhanced anticoagulant effect

Mefenamic acid – enhances anticoagulant effect

Progestogen – antagonism of anticoagulant effect

Pharmacodynamic properties

Synthetic anticoagulant of the coumarin series. It acts by inhibiting the formation of active clotting factors II, VII, IX and X. An effective prothrombin time (PT) can be achieved in 24–36 h post initial dose, max 36–48 h, and this therapeutic PT is maintained for 48 h after stopping drug

Continued

Fetal risk

Fetal teratogen, causes multiple disorders and malformations; should be stopped preconception or within 6 weeks' gestation (see above); haemorrhage in fetus and placenta in all trimesters; postnatal developmental delay

Breastfeeding

Excreted in breast milk in small amounts; theoretical risk of haemorrhage, especially with vitamin K deficiency, but considered safe if dose within therapeutic range

New medications being marketed that have similar pharmacotherapeutic properties to warfarin sodium are:

- **Pradaxa** (dabigatran etexilate mesilate) (Boehringer Ingelheim Ltd)
- **Xarelto** (rivaraxaban) (Bayer PLC).

These drugs require less frequent monitoring of clotting times. Currently there is no indication of their efficacy or safety during childbearing.

BP
Protamine sulphate

Proprietary
Prosulf® (Wockhardt UK Ltd)
Protamine sulphate (Sovereign Medical)
(Non-proprietary, see BNF for detail)

Group
Heparin antagonist

Uses/indications
Reversal of the actions of heparin

Type of drug
POM

Presentation
Ampoules

Dosage
See BNF and manufacturers' guidelines. *In brief:*
1 mg neutralizes 100 units heparin (mucus) or 80 units (lung) within 15 min of administration; if longer, less is required as heparin is rapidly excreted. Max dose 50 mg in 10 min. Should be monitored by activated partial prothrombin time (APPT) or other clotting test 5–10 min after administration; further doses may be required as protamine is cleared more rapidly than heparin, especially LMWH

Route of admin
Slow IV injection

Contraindications
Hypersensitivity to protamine; caution in those receiving protamine insulin preparation, i.e. isophane insulin, fish allergy

Side effects
Flushing, nausea, vomiting, hypotension, bradycardia; if overdosed then acts as an anticoagulant

Interactions
Caution in those receiving isophane insulins – hypersensitivity

Pharmacodynamic properties
A potent antidote to heparin but the precise mechanism is unknown. It is assumed that the strongly basic protamine combines with the strongly acid heparin to produce a stable salt that has no anticoagulant activity

Fetal risk
Insufficient information available – no animal or human studies have been carried out

Breastfeeding
No data available – as for fetal risk

BP
Phytomenadione (Vitamin K)

Proprietary
Konakion® MM 10 mg in 1 mL and Konakion MM
Paediatric 2 mg in 0.2 mL (Roche Products Ltd)

Group
Warfarin antagonist

Uses/indications
Prevention and treatment of haemorrhage

Type of drug
POM and Black Triangle
this medicine is monitored intensively by the CHM and
MHRA

Presentation
Ampoules

Dosage
Refer to manufacturers' guidelines:
ADULT: *Prophylaxis – Obstetric cholestasis and epilepsy;*
from 36 weeks of pregnancy (RCOG, 2009) recommend
10 mg daily especially when APPT is prolonged, or if
steatorrhoea is present
Life-threatening haemorrhage: 5 mg slow IV injection
plus plasma (factors II, IX, VII if available)
Less severe haemorrhage: withhold warfarin and consider
0.5–2 mg slow IV injection
repeat APPT levels 3 h post dose and if not responsive
then repeat dose – not more than 40 mg in 24 h
PAEDIATRIC: *Prophylaxis – Vitamin K deficiency bleeding:*
Healthy newborns of 36 weeks' gestation and older:
Either 1 mg administered by IM injection at birth or
soon after birth **or** 2 mg orally at birth or soon after
birth. The oral dose should be followed by a second
dose of 2 mg at 4–7 days
*Exclusively breast-fed babies who received oral Konakion at
birth*: In addition to the doses at birth and at 4–7 days, a
further 2 mg oral dose should be given 1 month after birth

Preterm neonates of less than 36 weeks' gestation weighing 2.5 kg or more, and term neonates at special risk: 1 mg IM or IV at birth or soon after birth, the size and frequency of further doses depending on coagulation status

Preterm neonates of less than 36 weeks' gestation weighing less than 2.5 kg: 0.4 mg/kg (equivalent to 0.04 mL/kg) IM or IV at birth or soon after birth. The frequency of further doses should depend on coagulation status

Haemorrhage: initial dose of 1 mg IV and further dose will depend on coagulation profile

Route of admin
Very slow IV injection, oral, IM

Contraindications
No data available

Side effects
Anaphylactoid reactions after intravenous injections of Konakion MM;, rarely, venous irritation or phlebitis

Interactions
Anticoagulants – antagonism of the anticoagulant effect

Pharmacodynamic properties
Synthetic vitamin K. Vitamin K is essential for the formation of prothrombin, factor VII, factor IX, and factor X. Without vitamin K there is a tendency to haemorrhage

Fetal risk
Poor placental transfer; no risk data available

Breastfeeding
Maternal doses – not enough information available to allow classification as safe drug. Large maternal doses of anticoagulants may require neonatal vitamin K prophylaxis

Low molecular weight heparin (LMWH) acts slightly differently to unfractionated heparin (UFH). It is essential to have an understanding of the coagulation cascade in order to understand how and why heparin is an anticoagulant. The advantage of LMWH over UFH is in its action: the actions of UFH are influenced by its binding to plasma protein, endothelial cell surfaces, macrophages and other acute-phase reactants in the anticoagulant cascade. LMWH has decreased binding to non-anticoagulant-related plasma proteins. The anticoagulant response is predictable and reproducible, with no need for laboratory monitoring, and it is given on a weight-adjusted basis. It has a high bioavailability of 90%, compared with 30% for UFH, and has a longer plasma half-life of 4–6 hours versus 0.5–1 hours for UFH. There is less inhibition of platelet function and potentially less bleeding risk, although this is unproven. There is a lower incidence of thrombocytopenia and thrombosis as there is less interaction with platelet factor 4 (http://chestjournal.chestpubs.org/content/119/1_suppl/64S.full).

Below are some of the LMWH and their dosages, properties, pregnancy and breastfeeding risks:

- OVERDOSE: protamine sulphate only partially neutralizes these drugs, so use with caution and consider the side effects of protamine carefully.

BP
Dalteparin sodium

Proprietary
Fragmin® (Pfizer Ltd)

Group
LMWH

Presentation
Single-dose syringe, ampoules, vials

Dosage
PE/DVT: S.C., depending on body weight: 69–82 kg, 15 000 units daily; 83 kg and over, 18 000 units daily oral anticoagulants can be used concomitantly until therapeutic range is achieved (usually 5 days)

Route of admin
S.C.

Pharmacodynamic properties
Porcine-derived sodium heparin and antithrombotic agent with the ability to potentiate the inhibition of Factor Xa and thrombin by antithrombin. This ability is relatively higher than disruption of the plasma clotting line (expressed as APTT); therefore, compared with UFH, dalteparin has fewer adverse effects on platelet function and adhesion, thus giving only minimal effects on primary haemostasis

Fetal risk
Does not pass the placenta; as for heparin

Breastfeeding
As for heparin

BP
Enoxoparin

Proprietary
Clexane® (Sanofi-Aventis)

Group
LMWH

Presentation
single dose syringe, vials

Dosage
PE/DVT: S.C. 1.5 mg/kg every 24 h for at least 5 days or until oral anticoagulation is established (150 units/kg daily)
NB: unlicensed indication for use during pregnancy for treatment of venous thromboembolism.
Prophylaxis: moderate risk 20 mg (2000 units) daily for 7–10 days
High risk: 40 mg (4000 units) daily
Medical clients: 40 mg (4000 units) daily for 6 days or until ambulant

Route of admin
S.C.

Pharmacodynamic properties
LMWH with antithrombotic activity. There is a greater rate of this than with UFH, and at the recommended dose it does not significantly alter platelet aggregation, the binding of fibrinogen to platelets, or global clotting tests such as APTT and PT time

Fetal risk
No evidence that enoxaparin crosses the placental barrier; evidence of risk in the second trimester but no information on the first and third trimesters. As there are no adequate controlled studies it is not advised for use unless there is no safe alternative

Breastfeeding
Excretion into breast milk is unlikely but manufacturer advises avoidance

---

BP
Tinzeparin sodium

Proprietary
Innohep® (Leo Laboratories Ltd)

Group
LMWH

Presentation
Single-dose syringe, ampoules

Dosage
Caution: can cause bronchospasm and shock in asthmatics
PE/DVT: S.C. 175 units/kg daily for 6 days or until oral anticoagulation is established after epidural/spinal anaesthesia; delay subsequent dose by at least 4 h

Route of admin
S.C.

Pharmacodynamic properties
Antithrombotic agent that acts by inhibiting the action of several activated coagulation factors, especially Factor Xa

> **Fetal risk**
> No transplacental transmission has been found in the second trimester, but studies in rats show low birthweight; therefore the manufacturer advises avoidance
>
> **Breastfeeding**
> No evidence of excretion found, but manufacturer advises avoidance

References and Recommended Reading

Baxter, K., 2011. Stockley's Drug Interaction Companion. Pharmaceutical Press, London.

Briggs, G., Freeman, R., Yaffe, S., 2008. Drugs in Pregnancy and Lactation: A Reference Guide to Fetal and Neonatal Risk, eighth ed. Lippincott Williams and Wilkins, Philadelphia.

Bubimschi, C., Weiner, C., 2010. Medication. In: James, D.K., Steer, P.J., Weiner, C.P., Gonik, B. (Eds.), High Risk Pregnancy: Management Options, fourth ed. Elsevier Saunders, London, pp. 579–598.

Farquharson, R.G., Greaves, M., 2010. Thromboembolic disease. In: James, D.K., Steer, P.J., Weiner, C.P., Gonik, B. (Eds.), High Risk Pregnancy: Management Options, fourth ed. Elsevier Saunders, London, pp. 453–462.

Hofmeyr, G.J., Neilson, J.P., Alfirevic, Z., Crowther, C., Duley, L., Gulmezoglu, M., Gyte, G.M., Hodnett, E.D., 2008. Pregnancy and Childbirth – A Cochrane Pocketbook. Wiley Cochrane Series, London.

Joint Formulary Committee, 2011. British National Formulary (BNF) 62. Pharmaceutical Press, London.

Jordan, S., 2010. Drugs affecting the coagulation process. In: Jordan, S. (Ed.), Pharmacology for Midwives: The Evidence Base for Safe Practice, second ed. Palgrave Macmillan, Basingstoke, pp. 199–220.

Koren, G., 2007. Medication Safety in Pregnancy and Breastfeeding: The Evidence Based A–Z Clinician's Pocket Guide. McGraw-Hill, New York.

Royal College of Obstetricians and Gynaecologists 2009. Thrombosis and Embolism During Pregnancy and the Puerperium: Reducing the Risk. Greentop guideline 37a. RCOG, London

Rubin, P.C., Ramsey, M., 2007. Prescribing in Pregnancy, fourth ed. BMJ Books/Blackwell Publishing, Oxford.

Schaefer, C., Peters, P.W.J., Miller, R.K. (Eds.), 2007. Drugs During Pregnancy and Lactation: Treatment Options and Risk Assessment, Academic Press/Elsevier, London.

SPC from the eMC, Clexane® injection, Sanofi Aventis, updated on the eMC 26/7/11.

SPC from the eMC, Fragmin® 7500–18,000 IU single dose syringes, Pfizer Ltd, updated on the eMC 5/7/11.

SPC from the eMC, Heparin Sodium® 1000 IU/mL; 5000 IU/mL; 25,000 IU/mL for injection, Wockhardt UK Ltd, updated on the eMC 22/3/11.

SPC from the eMC, Innohep® 10,000 IU/mL and 20,000 IU/mL syringe, Leo Laboratories Ltd, updated on the eMC 3/10/11.

SPC from the eMC, Konakion MM®, Paediatric Roche Products Ltd, updated on the eMC 1/2/11.

SPC from the eMC, Marevan® (Warfarin Sodium) 0.5 mg, 1 mg, 3 mg or 5 mg tablets, Goldshield Group Ltd, updated on the eMC 20/8/10.

SPC from the eMC, Prosulf® 10 mg/mL protamine sulphate injection, Wockhardt UK Ltd, updated on the eMC 27/9/10.

Volans, G., Wiseman, H., 2012. Drugs Handbook 2012–2013, thirty-third ed. Palgrave Macmillan, Basingstoke.

6

Anticonvulsants

Anticonvulsants are drugs used to arrest or prevent fits or seizures. The benefits of treatment should outweigh the risk to the fetus, and efforts should be made to use the single most effective drug, as teratogenicity increases with the number of drugs used. Pre-conceptual advice is strongly recommended.

This drug group inhibits the uptake of folic acid, and therefore any supplements given may need to be continued throughout pregnancy.

Magnesium sulphate is also an anticonvulsant used in the emergency treatment of eclampsia – see Chapter 25.

The student should be aware of:

- conditions that require anticonvulsant therapy
- local protocols for anticonvulsant therapy and specific medical conditions
- recognition of fits, seizures and convulsions
- resuscitative techniques and care of affected clients
- maternal and fetal sequelae of absorption of these preparations.

Interactions

Phenytoin

Alcohol – high intake increases plasma phenytoin levels; chronic abuse decreases serum levels

Analgesics – NSAIDs increase the plasma phenytoin concentration

Antacids – reduce the absorption of phenytoin; cimetidine decreases the metabolism of phenytoin and therefore increases its plasma concentration

Antibiotics – metronidazole increases the plasma phenytoin concentration; plasma concentration and antifolate effect increased by co-trimoxazole and trimethoprim

Anticoagulants – probably reduce the effect of warfarin

Antidepressants – tricyclics decrease the phenytoin plasma concentration and the convulsive threshold

Antiepileptics – two or more antiepileptics enhance toxicity; monitoring of plasma concentrations required

Antiemetics – stemetil and derivatives lower convulsive threshold

Antihypertensives – nifedipine increases phenytoin plasma concentration; the effect of nifedipine is reduced

Anxiolytics and hypnotics – diazepam can increase or decrease plasma phenytoin concentration

Corticosteroids – metabolism is increased, so effect is decreased

Contraceptives – metabolism of oral contraceptives is increased, so their effect is decreased

Vitamins – the plasma phenytoin concentration is lowered by folic acid; vitamin D supplements may be required.

Phenobarbital

Alcohol – increased sedative effect

Antibiotics – metabolism of metronidazole is increased, so the effect is decreased

Anticoagulants – metabolism of warfarin increased, so effect is decreased

Antidepressants – tricyclics decrease the plasma concentration and the convulsive threshold

Antiepileptics – as for phenytoin; requires dose monitoring

Antiemetics – as for phenytoin

Antihypertensives – effect of nifedipine reduced

Corticosteroids – as for phenytoin
Contraceptives – as for phenytoin
Folic acid – phenobarbital has antifolate effect

Sodium valproate

Analgesics – aspirin enhances effect
Antacids – cimetidine increases plasma levels of valproate
Antibiotics – erythromycin increases plasma levels of valproate
Antiemetics – as for phenytoin
Antiepileptics – with two or more, close monitoring is
    required
Anticoagulants – increased anticoagulant effect – monitoring
    of PT required
Cholestyramine – decreases absorption of valproate
Zidovudine – antagonism of the metabolism of zidovudine, so
    increased toxicity

Carbamazepine

Alcohol – enhanced CNS effects
Antidepressants – tricyclics have an accelerated metabolism,
    so decreased effect; monitoring required
Antiepileptics – plasma concentration effected by concomitant
    use, so careful plasma monitoring required
Anticoagulants – decreased anticoagulant effect of warfarin
Cimetidine – inhibits the metabolism of carbamazepine, so
    increases plasma concentration
Corticosteroids – carbamazepine increases the metabolism of
    both β-prednisolone and dexamethasone
Dextropropoxyphene – increases effect of carbamazepine
Erythromycin – increased plasma concentrations of
    carbamazepine
Nifedipine – decreased antiepileptic effect
OCP – decreased contraceptive effect
Tramadol – decreased effect of tramadol

BP
Sodium valproate

Proprietary
Epilim® (Sanofi-Aventis)
Sodium valproate (non-proprietary, see BNF for details)

Group
Anticonvulsant

Uses/indications
All forms of epilepsy

Type of drug
POM

Presentation
Tablets, solution, syrup, powder for reconstitution

Dosage
Oral: 600 mg–2.5 g/day in two divided doses
IV/IV infusion: same as oral but over 3–5 min

Route of admin
Oral, IV/IV infusion

Contraindications
Pregnancy and breastfeeding, hepatic or renal
impairment, SLE

Side effects
Gastrointestinal disturbances, nausea, ataxia, tremor,
weight gain, hair loss, hepatic impairment, disturbed
platelet function, pancreatitis; multiple therapy requires
care

Interactions
See start of chapter

Pharmacodynamic properties
Likely mode of action is potentiation of the inhibitory
action of GABA, through action on the further synthesis
or metabolism of GABA

Fetal risk
Spina bifida, neonatal bleeding, hepatotoxicity, fetal growth deficiency, hyperbilirubinaemia, fetal distress, craniofacial defects, urogenital defects, hypospadias up to 50%, retarded psychomotor development, digital abnormalities

Breastfeeding
Secreted in breast milk – in low doses appears safe; high doses – insufficient information to qualify as safe

---

BP
Phenytoin

Proprietary
Epanutin® (Pfizer Ltd)
Phenytoin (non-proprietary, see BNF for details)

Group
Anticonvulsant/antiepileptic

Uses/indications
Epilepsy, fits – not absence seizures, treatment of eclampsia

Type of drug
POM

Presentation
Capsules, tablets, suspension

Dosage
With or after food: maintenance doses 150–300 mg/day in 1–2 divided doses or as per protocol (plasma values need evaluation and observation)
IV: phenytoin sodium in treatment of eclampsia as per protocol

Route of admin
Oral, IV

Contraindications
Pregnancy and breastfeeding, hepatic impairment, hypersensitivity, shock

Continued **81**

Side effects
OVERDOSE: no known antidote – possibly removed from plasma by haemodialysis

Nausea, vomiting, headache, tremor, insomnia; prolonged usage – hirsutism, coarse facies, acne, gingival hyperplasia, confusion

Interactions
See start of chapter

Pharmacodynamic properties
Appears to stabilize rather than raise seizure threshold, and to prevent the spread of seizure activity rather than abolish the primary focus of seizure discharge. The mechanism is not fully understood but may include:

- a reduction in sodium conductance by enhancing its extrusion, thereby preventing potential seizure activity
- enhancing the action of GABA inhibition and reducing excitatory synaptic transmission
- presynaptic reduction of calcium entry and block of release of neurotransmitters

Fetal risk
In trimesters 1 and 3 teratogen; maternal folic acid supplements should be given under medical supervision; increased risk of haemorrhage in the neonate – prophylaxis with vitamin K recommended

Breastfeeding
Secreted in breast milk, some minor effects noted, mother and child should be monitored, manufacturer advises avoidance unless necessary

---

BP
Phenobarbital

Proprietary
Phenobarbital (Actavis UK Ltd)

Group
Antiepileptic – barbiturate

Uses/indications
Epilepsy – not absence seizures

Type of drug
POM, CD

Presentation
Tablets

Dosage
Oral: 50–200 mg q.d.s. to a max 600 mg/day (monitoring for plasma concentration of 15–40 mcg/mL (65–170 micromoles/L))
IM: 50–200 mg q.d.s. to a max 600 mg/day (plasma monitoring is less useful as tolerance occurs from prolonged treatment regimens)

Route of admin
Oral, IM, IV injection

Contraindications
Pregnancy, breastfeeding, impaired hepatic or renal function, respiratory depression

Side effects
Tolerance develops, drowsiness, neural depression, allergic skin reactions, overdose

Interactions
See start of chapter

Pharmacodynamic properties
A long-acting barbiturate that is an effective anticonvulsant. It appears to raise/elevate the seizure threshold and limit the spread of seizure activity. The mechanism is unknown but may involve an increase in the GABA synergic systems

Fetal risk
In trimesters 1 and 3, a teratogen, particularly neural tube defects, hypoprothrombinaemia and withdrawal in infants with maternal treatment late in pregnancy; concomitant administration with other antiepileptics has been linked to haemorrhagic disease of the newborn within the first 24 h of life – prophylaxis with vitamin K is recommended

Continued

Breastfeeding
Avoid where possible, as drowsiness in infant and other minor effects reported. Mother and baby need to be monitored

---

BP
Carbamazepine

Proprietary
Tegretol® (Novartis Pharmaceuticals UK Ltd)
Carbamazepine (non-proprietary, see BNF for details)

Group
Anticonvulsant

Uses/indications
Epilepsy, generalized seizures and partial seizures, not absence seizures or myoclonic seizures (trigeminal neuralgia)

Type of drug
POM

Presentation
Tablets, suppositories, liquid, chewtabs

Dosage
Oral: initially 100–200 mg once or twice daily/day, usually 0.8–1.2 g in evenly divided doses, increased until best response
P.R.: when oral not available – 125 mg is considered equivalental to 100 mg

Route of admin
Oral, P.R.

Contraindications
Pregnancy, breastfeeding, history of bone marrow depression, hepatic/renal impairment, blood hepatic or skin disorders, glaucoma, sensitivity to either carbamazepine or structurally similar drugs, use of tricyclic or MAOI drugs

Side effects
Side effects are common and appear dose related, resolving spontaneously or after transient dose reduction; gastrointestinal disturbances, drowsiness, headaches, visual disturbances, rashes, blood disorders, including thrombocytopenia, hepatic/renal disorders

Interactions
See start of chapter

Pharmacodynamic properties
Exact mechanism unknown, but thought to stabilize hyperexcited nerve membranes, inhibiting repetitive neuronal discharges and reducing excitatory impulses. It also reduces glutamate release and blockades sodium channels, thereby stabilizing neuronal membranes and action potentials

Fetal risk
Animal studies show an increase in mortality if taken during organogenesis; later administration caused growth retardation in rat fetuses – women who take carbamazepine should be counselled for risk and given antenatal screening, and the benefits of administration should be weighed against the risks. There is also a theorctical risk of HDN in the neonate, therefore prophylactic vitamin K is recommended

Breastfeeding
Excreted but considered safe in common doses, although manufacturer recommends observation for side effects

References and Recommended Reading

Baxter, K., 2011. Stockley's Drug Interaction Companion. Pharmaceutical Press, London.

Bewley, C., 2011. Medical disorders of pregnancy. In: Macdonald, S., Magill-Cuerden, J. (Eds.), Mayes' Midwifery, fourteenth ed. Baillière Tindall/Elsevier, Edinburgh, pp. 771–786.

Briggs, G., Freeman, R., Yaffe, S., 2008. Drugs in Pregnancy and Lactation: A Reference Guide to Fetal and Neonatal Risk, eighth ed. Lippincott Williams and Wilkins, Philadelphia.

Bubimschi, C., Weiner, C., 2010. Medication. In: James, D.K., Steer, P.J., Weiner, C.P., Gonik, B. (Eds.), High Risk Pregnancy: Management Options, fourth ed. Elsevier Saunders, London, pp. 579–598.

Carbuapoma, J.R., Tomlinson, M.W., Levina, S.R., 2010. Neurological complications. In: James, D.K., Steer, P.J., Weiner, C.P., Gonik, B. (Eds.), High Risk Pregnancy: Management Options, fourth ed. Elsevier Saunders, London, pp. 861–892.

Hofmeyr, G.J., Neilson, J.P., Alfreirevic, Z., Crowther, C., Duley, L., Gulmezoglu, M., Gyte, G.M., Hodnett, E.D., 2008. Pregnancy and Childbirth – A Cochrane Pocketbook. Wiley Cochrane Series, London.

Joint Formulary Committee, 2011. British National Formulary (BNF) 62. Pharmaceutical Press, London.

Koren, G., 2007. Medication Safety in Pregnancy and Breastfeeding: The Evidence Based A–Z Clinician's Pocket Guide. McGraw-Hill, New York.

Paediatric Formulary Committee, 2011. BNF for Children 2011–2012. Pharmaceutical Press, London.

Rubin, P.C., Ramsey, M., 2007. Prescribing in Pregnancy, fourth ed. BMJ Books/Blackwell Publishing, Oxford.

Sassarini, J., Clerk, N., Jordan, S., 2010. Epilepsy in pregnancy. In: Jordan, S. (Ed.), Pharmacology for Midwives: The Evidence Base for Safe Practice, second ed. Palgrave Macmillan, Basingstoke, pp. 361–376.

Schaefer, C., Peters, P.W.J., Miller, R.K. (Eds.), 2007. Drugs During Pregnancy and Lactation: Treatment Options and Risk Assessment, Academic Press/Elsevier, London.

SPC from the eMC, Epanutin®, capsules, ready mixed, parenteral, Pfizer Limited, updated on the eMC 17/10/11.

SPC from the eMC, Epilim®, Sanofi Aventis, updated on the eMC 28/7/11.

SPC from the eMC, Phenobarbitol 30 mg and 60 mg tablets, Actavis UK Ltd, updated on the eMC 7/1/11.

SPC from the eMC, Tegretol® Chewtabs 100 mg, 200 mg, Tegretol® tablets 100 mg, 200 mg, 400 mg, suppositories 125 mg and 250 mg, Novartis Pharmaceuticals UK Ltd, updated on the eMC 8/12/09.

Volans, G., Wiseman, H., 2012. Drugs Handbook 2012–2013, thirtythird ed. Palgrave Macmillan, Basingstoke.

7

Antidepressants and Treatments for Mental Health Conditions

Antidepressants

These are preparations that aim to restore the balance of neurotransmitter substances in the brain, a deficiency of which is thought to contribute to depression. They are usually selective serotonin reuptake inhibitors (SSRIs), monoamine oxidase inhibitors (MAOIs) or tricyclic antidepressants.

St John's wort (*Hypericum perforatum*) is a popular herbal remedy for mild depression. However, it does interact with many prescribed medications including antidepressants, and its use should be carefully monitored and advice sought from a medical practitioner.

Antimania Drugs

These are medications used to control acute and episodes of mania or hypomania. Benzodiazepines are also used to treat behavioural disturbances.

The student should be aware of:

■ the clinical signs and progression of antenatal and postnatal depression (PND)

■ the maternal and fetal sequelae of therapy

- the local availability of counselling and facilities for treatment
- the consequences for lack of either diagnosis or treatment of depression
- the research into PND and its relation to hypothyroidism in certain cases.

CAUTION: The authors recommend that drugs in this group should be investigated individually, as psychiatry is a specialized field and most antidepressants require comprehensive monitoring in pregnancy and during breastfeeding.

BP
Dothiepin hydrochloride (Dosulepin)

Proprietary
Prothiaden® (Teofarma)
Dothiepin hydrochloride (non-proprietary, see BNF for details)

Group
Antidepressant – tricyclic

Uses/indications
Depression where sedation is required, e.g. postnatal depression

Type of drug
POM

Presentation
Capsules (25 mg), tablets (75 mg)

Dosage
Oral: 75 mg daily (divided or single) increased to 150–225 mg daily

Route of admin
Oral

Contraindications
Recent myocardial infarction, mania

Side effects
Dry mouth, sedation, blurred vision, cardiovascular disturbances, blood sugar changes

Interactions

Alcohol – avoid – enhanced sedative effect
Antidepressants – CNS excitation, hypertension with MAOIs – avoid for 2 weeks after stopping MAOI
Antiepileptics – convulsive threshold and tricyclic plasma concentration are lowered
Antihistamines – increased antimuscarinic and sedative effect, ventricular arrhythmias with terfenadine and astemizole
Antihypertensives – increases hypotensive effect
Contraceptives – antagonizes effect of antidepressants, but side effects increase the plasma concentration of tricyclics

Pharmacodynamic properties
Tricyclic antidepressant that acts to increase transmitter levels at central synapses; this produces a clinical antidepressant effect. The inhibition of the re-uptake of noradrenaline (norepinephrine) and 5-hydroxytryptamine (5HT) and the uptake of dopamine produces adaptive changes in the brain that enhance the antidepressant effects

Fetal risk
Higher fetal toxicity than SSRIs; tachycardia, irritability, muscle spasms and neonatal convulsions

Breastfeeding
Amount secreted too small to be harmful in short-term use; accumulation may cause sedation and respiratory depression

BP
Fluoxetine

Proprietary
Prozac® (Eli Lilly & Co. Ltd)

Group
Antidepressant – SSRI

Uses/indications
Depressive illness, bulimia nervosa, obsessive–compulsive disorder

Type of drug
POM

Presentation
Capsules, liquid (5 mL = 20 mg)

Dosage
20 mg daily (varies according to condition)

Route of admin
Oral

Contraindications
Mania, cardiac disease, epilepsy, hepatic/renal impairment, pregnancy, breastfeeding, concomitant use of MAOI

Side effects
Gastrointestinal disturbances, hypersensitivity, anxiety, palpitations, tremors, hair loss, confusion, hypotension, drowsiness, blood disorders, liver disturbances, suicidal thoughts

Interactions
Alcohol – alcohol and SSRIs are inadvisable
Antidepressants – enhance toxicity and levels require monitoring
Antiepileptics – carbamazepine and phenytoin enhance toxicity and levels require monitoring
Anticoagulants – warfarin – increased bleeding time, levels need monitoring
Antihypertensives – enhanced hypotensive effect
Pharmacodynamic properties
Selective inhibitor of serotonin reuptake

Fetal risk
First trimester – cardiovascular anomalies; third trimester – risk (5 per 1000 pregnancies) of persistent pulmonary hypertension in the newborn (PPHN); manufacturer advises use only if the benefits outweigh the risks post-birth: these effects have been reported in neonates – irritability, tremor, hypotonia, persistent crying, difficulty in sucking or in sleeping

Breastfeeding
Significant amounts are excreted into milk and considered moderately safe; manufacturer advises avoidance unless the benefits outweigh the risks

---

BP
Progesterone

Proprietary
Cyclogest® (Actavis UK Ltd)

Group
Hormones – progesterone

Uses/indications
Premenstrual syndrome, puerperal depression – although there is no convincing evidence of physiological effectiveness, may be used for the alleviation of PND

Type of drug
POM

Presentation
Pessaries (for vaginal or rectal use)

Dosage
200–400 mg

Route of admin
P.R., P.V.

Contraindications
Diabetes, breastfeeding, hypertension, renal, hepatic or cardiac disease

Continued

Side effects
Acne, urticaria, fluid retention, weight change, gastrointestinal disturbances, changes in libido

Interactions
None known

Pharmacodynamic properties
Progestational steroid

Fetal risk
High doses can be teratogenic in the first trimester

Breastfeeding
High doses can inhibit or suppress lactation

BP
Lithium carbonate/Lithium citrate

Proprietary
Priadel® 200 mg and 400 mg prolonged release tablets
Priadel® Liquid (Sanofi-Aventis)
Camcolit® 250 mg and 400 mg (Norgine Ltd)

Group
Antimania drug

Uses/indications
Management of acute manic or hypomanic episodes, recurrent depressive disorders where treatment with other antidepressants has been unsuccessful, prophylaxis for bipolar affective disorders, control of aggressive behaviour or intentional self-harm

Type of drug
POM

Presentation
(Prolonged release) tablet, liquid

Dosage
Priadel® prolonged release tablets – 400–1200 mg in single dose, morning or before bed
CAUTION: regular monitoring of serum lithium levels, monitoring of well-being and planned multi-professional care plans are recommended in providing care for women on lithium medications (NICE, 2007)

Route of admin
Oral

Contraindications
Diabetes, untreated hypothyroidism, breastfeeding, hypertension, renal, hepatic or cardiac disease

Side effects
Acne, urticaria, fluid retention, weight change, gastrointestinal disturbances, changes in libido

Interactions
Antibiotics – reduce renal clearance, e.g. metronidazole, tetracyclines, co-trimazole, trimethoprim
ACE inhibitors, diuretics, NSAIDs, steroids – increase lithium concentrations (risk of toxicity)
Sodium-based products, caffeine, theophylline, diuretics, urea – decrease lithium concentrations
Antipsychotics (clozapine, haloperidol), carbamazepine, phenytoin, methyldopa, tricyclic antidepressants, calcium channel blockers, SSRIs, NSAIDs – neurotoxicity, even if lithium levels in normal range
NB: lithium toxicity can also occur when other health issues arise, e.g. infection, pregnancy-onset conditions, physical or psychological changes

Pharmacodynamic properties
Mood-stabilizing agent; lithium is an alkali metal as lithium carbonate or lithium citrate; modifies the production and turnover of certain neurotransmitters, particularly serotonin, and may also block dopamine receptors; modifies concentrations of some electrolytes, particularly calcium and magnesium; and may reduce thyroid activity

Fetal risk
High doses can be teratogenic in the first trimester –
cardiac anomalies especially. Ebstein anomaly, and
other malformations have been reported

Breastfeeding
Is secreted in breast milk and there have been case
reports of neonates showing signs of lithium toxicity

BP
Methadone

Proprietary
Methadone® 5 mg/mL oral solution (Pinewood
Healthcare)
Methadone (non-proprietary, see BNF for details)

Group
Substance dependence

Uses/indications
Management of opioid dependence under the
supervision of an appropriate physician

Type of drug
POM

Presentation
Clear or light amber solution for oral use

Dosage
Calculated for individual and serum monitoring
NB: long half-life in system

Route of admin
Oral – not for dilution or injection unless specified by
manufacturer

Contraindications

Hypersensitivity, acute asthma, head injury, acute alcoholism, concurrent use of MAOIs

Pregnancy/labour – not recommended as may cause neonatal respiratory depression, withdrawal symptoms in the neonate

Manufacturers advise caution in hypothyroidism, adrenal disease, inflammatory bowel disease

Side effects

Overdose: symptoms/signs in methadone overdose are essentially as for morphine, although methadone has a greater respiratory depressive effect and a lesser sedative effect than an equivalent dose of morphine

Toxicity: highly variable dosages, regular use leading to tolerance. Pulmonary oedema is a common effect of overdose; dose-related histamine-releasing property of methadone may cause urticaria and pruritus; may lead to an increase in intracranial pressure

Interactions

Naloxone (opioid antagonist) – counteracts the effects of methadone and induces abstinence

CNS depressants – may result in increased respiratory depression, hypotension, strong sedation or coma. Slow tolerance development; every dose increase may after 1–2 weeks give rise to symptoms of respiratory depression. Dose adjustments must be monitored carefully

Peristalsis inhibition – e.g. loperamide and methadone may result in severe constipation and increase the CNS depressant effects

Antidepressants (paroxetine, sertraline) or antibiotics (erythromycin, clarithromycin) – may cause changes to cardiac contractility (QT)

MAOIs – CNS inhibition, serious hypotonia and/or apnoea 2 weeks after cessation of treatment

Opioid analgesics – delay gastric emptying

Continued

Pharmacodynamic properties

Methadone is an opioid analgesic similar to morphine and is highly addictive; less sedative effect than morphine. It acts on the CNS system and smooth muscle via specific opiate receptor sites in the brain, spinal cord and nervous system

Methadone is an opioid agonist with actions predominantly at the μ receptor

Fetal risk

Limited data in humans show no increased risk of congenital abnormalities

Withdrawal symptoms/respiratory depression may occur in neonates of mothers treated with methadone chronically during pregnancy

Generally advisable not to detoxify the patient, especially after the 20th week of pregnancy, but to administer maintenance treatment with methadone

Methadone should be withheld just before and during birth because of the risk of neonatal respiratory depression

Breastfeeding

Excreted in breast milk; average milk/plasma ratio is 0.8; manufacturer recommends the benefits must be weighed against the risks to the infant

References and Recommended Reading

Baxter, K., 2011. Stockley's Drug Interaction Companion. Pharmaceutical Press, London.

Briggs, G., Freeman, R., Yaffe, S., 2008. Drugs in Pregnancy and Lactation: A Reference Guide to Fetal and Neonatal Risk, eighth ed. Lippincott Williams and Wilkins, Philadelphia.

Centre for Maternal and Child Enquiries, 2011. Saving Mothers' Lives, Reviewing Maternal Deaths to Make Motherhood Safer: 2006–2008. The 8th Report of the Confidential Enquiries into Maternal Deaths in the United Kingdom. Available from: http://www.oaa-anaes.ac.uk/assets/_managed/editor/File/Reports/2006-2008%20CEMD.pdf [accessed 2 March 2012].

Gutteridge, K., 2011. Maternal mental health and psychological problems. In: Macdonald, S., Magill-Cuerden, J. (Eds.), Mayes' Midwifery, fourteenth ed. Baillière Tindall/Elsevier, Edinburgh, pp. 939–952.

Haskett, R., 2010. Psychiatric illness. In: James, D.K., Steer, P.J., Weiner, C.P., Gonik, B. (Eds.), High Risk Pregnancy: Management Options, fourth ed. Elsevier Saunders, London, pp. 997–1110.

Joint Formulary Committee, 2011. British National Formulary (BNF) 62. Pharmaceutical Press, London.

Jordan, S., Hardy, B., 2010. Drugs and mental health. In: Jordan, S. (Ed.), Pharmacology for Midwives: The Evidence Base for Safe Practice, second ed. Palgrave Macmillan, Basingstoke, pp. 377–394.

Koren, G., 2007. Medication Safety in Pregnancy and Breastfeeding: The Evidence Based A–Z Clinician's Pocket Guide. McGraw-Hill, New York.

National Institute for Health and Clinical Excellence (NICE), 2007. Antenatal and Postnatal Mental Health. CG45. NICE, London.

Price, S. (Ed.), 2007. Mental Health in Pregnancy and Childbirth, Churchill Livingstone/Elsevier, Edinburgh.

Prothiaden® tablets 75 mg, Teofarma, updated in the BNF 62, 2011.

Rubin, P.C., Ramsey, M., 2007. Prescribing in Pregnancy, fourth ed. BMJ Books/Blackwell Publishing, Oxford.

Schaefer, C., Peters, P.W.J., Miller, R.K. (Eds.), 2007. Drugs During Pregnancy and Lactation: Treatment Options and Risk Assessment, Academic Press/Elsevier, London.

SPC from the eMC, Camcolit® 250 mg & 400 mg, Norgine Ltd, updated on the eMC 1/9/11.

SPC from the eMC, Cyclogest®, Actavis UK Ltd, updated on the eMC 16/7/07.

SPC from the eMC, Methadone® 5 mg/mL oral solution, Pinewood Healthcare, updated on the eMC 8/11/11.

SPC from the eMC, Priadel® 200 mg & 400 mg prolonged release tablets, and Priadel® Liquid, Sanofi-Aventis, updated on the eMC 1/12/11.

SPC from the eMC, Prozac®, Eli Lilly & Co. Ltd, updated on the eMC 13/10/11.

Volans, G., Wiseman, H., 2012. Drugs Handbook 2012–2013, thirtythird ed. Palgrave Macmillan, Basingstoke.

8

Antiemetics

These are drugs used to prevent or lessen nausea and vomiting. Some of these preparations may also be antipsychotics or antihistamines.

The student should be aware of:

- the actions of analgesics on the cerebral cortex
- the results of administration of the antipsychotic antiemetics, i.e. their potentiating effects
- the appropriateness of treatment using antiemetics, especially in early pregnancy.

BP
Prochlorperazine

Proprietary
Prochlorperazine 5 mg tablets (Actavis UK Ltd); 12.5 mg/mL injection (Goldshield Group Ltd); Stemetil® tablets, injection and syrup (Sanofi-Aventis) (non-proprietary, see BNF for details)

Group
Antiemetic – antipsychotic

Uses/indications
Prophylaxis with the use of opioid analgesic, with excessive emesis

Type of drug
POM

Presentation
Ampoules, tablets

Dosage
IM: 12.5 mg 6–8-hrly
Oral: initially 20 mg then 10 mg after 2 h
Prevention of emesis: 5–10 mg b.d. or t.d.s.
Migraine or labyrinthitis: 5 mg t.d.s.

Route of admin
IM, oral, P.R.

Contraindications
Pregnancy, myasthenia gravis, cardiovascular and respiratory disease, epilepsy, phaeochromocytoma, liver or renal dysfunction, hypothyroidism

Side effects
Can cause prolonged labour and should be withheld until 3–4 cm dilation, drowsiness, pallor, hypothermia, extrapyramidal effects, postural hypotension with tachycardia, liver dysfunction

Interactions
Alcohol – increases the sedative effect, particularly respiratory depression
Antacids – interfere with the absorption of oral Stemetil
Anaesthetics – increases their hypertensive effect
Antiepileptics – phenobarbital – decreases plasma concentrations but is not thought to be clinically significant
Antihistamines – increased risk of ventricular arrhythmias with terfenadine
Antihypertensives – with methyldopa there is an increased risk of extrapyramidal effects

Pharmacodynamic properties
A potent phenothiazine neuroleptic used in nausea and vomiting, and in schizophrenia, acute mania and the management of anxiety

Continued

Fetal risk
In the first trimester there are reports of congenital
defects associated with repeated use even at low doses,
but single or occasional low doses appear safe;
extrapyramidal symptoms in the neonate, lethargy and
tremor, low APGARs, paradoxical hyperexcitability

Breastfeeding
Amount probably too small to be excreted but avoid
unless absolutely necessary; the manufacturer
recommends against therapy during breastfeeding

BP
Metoclopramide hydrochloride

Proprietary
Maxolon® (Amdipharm PLC)

Group
Antiemetic

Uses/indications
Nausea, vomiting

Type of drug
POM

Presentation
Tablets, ampoules, infusion, oral suspension

Dosage
10–30mg daily in divided doses

Route of admin
IM, oral, IVI or slow IV

Contraindications
Hepatic and renal impairment; may cause hypertension
in phaeochromocytoma; caution in epilepsy

Side effects
Extrapyramidal effects, hyperprolactinaemia

Interactions
Analgesics – increases the absorption of aspirin and
paracetamol, thereby enhancing their effect

Opioid analgesics – antagonize the effect on gastrointestinal activity.
SSRIs – use with care

Pharmacodynamic properties
Action of metoclopramide is closely associated with the parasympathetic nervous control of the upper gastrointestinal (GI) tract. It encourages normal peristaltic action and is indicated in conditions where disturbed GI motility is an underlying factor

Fetal risk
Use with caution specifically in first trimester; there is no information on the long-term evaluation of infants exposed in utero

Breastfeeding
Use with caution as there is a theoretical risk of potent CNS effects

BP
Cyclizine

Proprietary
Valoid® (Amdipharm PLC)

Group
Anticholinerqic – antiemetic

Uses/indications
Prevention and treatment of nausea and vomiting

Type of drug
POM

Presentation
Tablets, ampoules

Dosage
Oral: 50 mg – max t.d.s
IM or IV: 50 mg can be t.d.s.
Post-op: slow IV injection 20 min before the end of surgery

Continued

Route of admin
Oral, IM, IV

Contraindications
Hypersensitivity to cyclizine, cardiac disease

Side effects
Hypotension, fall in cardiac output, urticaria, rash, drowsiness, oropharyngeal dryness, tachycardia, blurred vision, urinary retention, constipation

Interactions
Alcohol – enhances the effect of cyclizine
Analgesics – enhances soporific effect of pethidine
Anticholinergics – concomitant use gives enhanced effects
CNS suppressants – enhances the effect of cyclizine

Pharmacodynamic properties
A histamine H_1-receptor antagonist, cyclizine has a low incidence of drowsiness but has antiemetic and anticholinergic properties. The exact mechanism is unknown, but it is thought to act to increase lower oesophageal sphincter tone, and it may also have an inhibitory effect on the emetic centre located in the midbrain

Fetal risk
Manufacturer advises that animal studies indicate teratogenicity

Breastfeeding
No data available from controlled studies in breastfeeding women, but considered moderately safe

References and Recommended Reading

Baxter, K., 2011. Stockley's Drug Interaction Companion. Pharmaceutical Press, London.

Briggs, G., Freeman, R., Yaffe, S., 2008. Drugs in Pregnancy and Lactation: A Reference Guide to Fetal and Neonatal Risk, eighth ed. Lippincott Williams and Wilkins, Philadelphia.

Bubimschi, C., Weiner, C., 2010. Medication. In: James, D.K., Steer, P.J., Weiner, C.P., Gonik, B. (Eds.), High Risk Pregnancy: Management Options, fourth ed. Elsevier Saunders, London, pp. 579–598.

Joint Formulary Committee, 2011. British National Formulary (BNF) 62. Pharmaceutical Press, London.

Jordan, S., 2010. Antiemetics. In: Jordan, S. (Ed.), Pharmacology for Midwives: The Evidence Base for Safe Practice, second ed. Palgrave Macmillan, Basingstoke, pp. 131–147.

Koren, G., 2007. Medication Safety in Pregnancy and Breastfeeding: The Evidence Based A–Z Clinician's Pocket Guide. McGraw-Hill, New York.

Rubin, P.C., Ramsey, M., 2007. Prescribing in Pregnancy, fourth ed. BMJ Books/Blackwell Publishing, Oxford.

Schaefer, C., Peters, P.W.J., Miller, R.K. (Eds.), 2007. Drugs During Pregnancy and Lactation: Treatment Options and Risk Assessment, Academic Press/Elsevier, London.

SPC from the eMC, Maxolon® tablets 10 mg, injection 10 mg/2mL, Amdipharm PLC, updated on the eMC 31/1/11.

SPC from the eMC, Prochlorperazine injection B.P. 12.5 mg/mL, 1 mL & 2 mL, Goldshield Group Ltd, updated on the eMC 21/10/10.

SPC from the eMC, Prochlorperazine 5 mg tablets, Actavis UK Ltd, updated on the eMC 21/2/12.

SPC from the eMC, Stemetil® 5 mg tablets, Sanofi-Aventis, updated on the eMC 21/8/12.

SPC from the eMC, Valoid® 50 mg injection, Amdipharm Plc, updated on the eMC 13/4/10.

Volans, G., Wiseman, H., 2012. Drugs Handbook 2012–2013, thirtythird ed. Palgrave Macmillan, Basingstoke.

9

Antifungals

These are drugs used to combat fungal infections. They can be ingested or applied topically, depending on the infection.

The student should be aware of:

- common fungal infections in pregnancy and postnatal care
- the physiology and pathophysiology that allow these infections to flourish
- the appropriateness of the antifungal treatment prescribed.

| **BP** |
| Nystatin |

| **Proprietary** |
| Nystan® (E.R. Squibb and Sons Ltd) |
| Nystaform® cream (Typharm Ltd) |
| |
| **Group** |
| Antifungal |
| |
| **Uses/indications** |
| Candidiasis in the mouth, oesophagus or intestinal tract |
| |
| **Type of drug** |
| POM |
| |
| **Presentation** |
| Oral suspension (yellow), cream (light yellow) |
| |
| **Dosage** |
| **Adult:** oral – 500 000 units q.d.s. for 7 days, i.e. 5 mL suspension (contains sugar); cream –100 000 units/g 2–3 times per day to affected skin |
| **Paediatric:** oral – 100 000 units q.d.s. for 7 days, i.e. 1 mL suspension (contains sugar) |

Route of admin
Oral

Contraindications
Hypersensitivity to constituents

Side effects
Nausea, vomiting, hypersensitivity

Interactions
No data available

Pharmacodynamic properties
Antifungal that is not absorbed by the gastrointestinal tract, skin or vagina, and that inhibits growth of microbes, mostly yeasts and yeast-like fungi, e.g. *Candida albicans*

Fetal risk
No reports of complications after administration in pregnancy

Breastfeeding
Not known to be secreted in breast milk; manufacturers recommend caution

---

BP
Clotrimazole

Proprietary
Canesten® (Bayer plc), Clotrimazole (non-proprietary, see BNF for details)
Canesten® Oral Capsule (Fluconazole 150 mg) (Bayer plc); Diflucan™ 150 mg capsule (Pfizer Limited)

Group
Antifungal

Uses/indications
Candidiasis

Type of drug
POM, GSL, Pharmacy only (oral)

Continued

Presentation
Cream (topical – internal and external), pessaries (vaginal)

Dosage
See manufacturers' instructions

Route of admin
P.V. and topically to the external vulval area
Oral – not recommended during pregnancy or breastfeeding – see manufacturers' information

Contraindications
Hypersensitivity

Side effects
Occasional local irritation

Interactions
Antifungals – may reduce the efficacy of other drugs used in fungal disease, e.g. nystatin
Contraceptives – may affect latex condoms and diaphragms

Pharmacodynamic properties
Broad-spectrum antifungal effective against proliferating fungi, e.g. yeast, mould, dermatophytes, and others. The antimycotic effect against the cell wall releases hydrogen peroxide and causes cell death

Fetal risk
No adverse effects; no epidemiological data available, despite use over time

Breastfeeding
Considered safe as minimal absorption

References and Recommended Reading

Baxter, K., 2011. Stockley's Drug Interaction Companion. Pharmaceutical Press, London.

Briggs, G., Freeman, R., Yaffe, S., 2008. Drugs in Pregnancy and Lactation: A Reference Guide to Fetal and Neonatal Risk, eighth ed. Lippincott Williams and Wilkins, Philadelphia.

Joint Formulary Committee, 2011. British National Formulary (BNF) 62. Pharmaceutical Press, London.

Jordan, S., 2010. Pharmacology for Midwives: The Evidence Base for Safe Practice, second ed. Palgrave Macmillan, Basingstoke.

Koren, G., 2007. Medication Safety in Pregnancy and Breastfeeding: The Evidence Based A–Z Clinician's Pocket Guide. McGraw-Hill, New York.

Nystaform® cream 100,000 units/g, Typharm Ltd, updated in the BNF 62, 2011. Available: http://www.typharm.com/docs/Nystaform_SPC.pdf [accessed 24 March 2012].

Rubin, P.C., Ramsey, M., 2007. Prescribing in Pregnancy, fourth ed. BMJ Books/Blackwell Publishing, Oxford.

Schaefer, C., Peters, P.W.J., Miller, R.K. (Eds.), 2007. Drugs During Pregnancy and Lactation: Treatment Options and Risk Assessment, Academic Press/Elsevier, London.

SPC from the eMC, Canestan® antifungal cream, Bayer plc, updated on the eMC 21/7/10.

SPC from the eMC, Canesten® oral capsule (fluconazole 150 mg), Bayer plc, updated on the eMC 21/12/11.

SPC from the eMC, Canestan® vaginal pessary 100 mg, 200 mg and 500 mg, Bayer plc, updated on the eMC 20/9/10.

SPC from the eMC, Diflucan™ 150 mg capsule, Pfizer Ltd, updated on the eMC 25/1/12.

SPC from the eMC, Nystan® oral suspension (ready mixed) (100,000 IU/mL), E.R. Squibb & Sons Ltd, updated on the eMC 16/2/10.

Volans, G., Wiseman, H., 2012. Drugs Handbook 2012–2013, thirtythird ed. Palgrave Macmillan, Basingstoke.

10

Antihistamines

The term 'antihistamine' refers to H_2 receptor antagonists and are subdivided into sedating antihistamines and non-sedating antihistamines. Uses include:

- Antiemetics for nausea and vomiting (see Chapter 8)
- Emergency treatment (anaphylactic shock)
- Allergy relief
- Cholestasis of pregnancy
- Premedication and sedation
- Insomnia
- Relief of colds and coughs.

Histamine is present in animal tissues and some release occurs after injury, but also after an allergic reaction, and gives rise to urticaria, asthma, hay fever and ultimately anaphylaxis. Antihistamines are palliative agents because they neither destroy nor prevent the release of histamine, but act by blocking access to histamine receptor sites and thereby inhibiting an allergic reaction. Antihistamines are usually thought of as being taken orally, but they can be injected; for example, chlorpheniramine and promazine are used as adjuncts to adrenaline (epinephrine) in the treatment of anaphylaxis (see Chapter 25). They can also be used intranasally, intraocularly and topically.

The student should be aware of:

- the physiology related to allergic response
- the most common factors causing allergic response
- recognition of and treatment for anaphylactic shock
- interactions of drug therapy that may produce an allergic response.

Midwives can administer 'adrenaline 1:1000' for anaphylaxis under the Midwives' Exemptions (NMC, 2011).

BP
Chlorpheniramine maleate

Proprietary
Piriton® (GlaxoSmithKline Consumer Healthcare)
Chlorpheniramine maleate (non-proprietary, see BNF for details)

Group
Antihistamine – sedative

Uses/indications
Symptomatic control of all allergic conditions responsive to antihistamines, including hay fever, vasomotor rhinitis, urticaria, angioneurotic oedema, food allergy, drug and serum reactions, insect bites
Symptomatic relief of itch associated with chickenpox
anaphylaxis – see Chapter 25

Type of drug
POM, GSL

Presentation
Tablets (4 mg), syrup (2 mg/5 mL), ampoules (10 mg/mL)

Dosage
General use: oral 4 mg 4–6-hrly to a max 24 mg daily
IM or IV over 1 min, 10 mg, repeated if required up to max 4 doses in 24 h
Emergency use: see Chapter 25

Route of admin
Oral, IM, IV (see Chapter 25 on emergency drugs)

Contraindications
Epilepsy, hepatic disease, asthma, patients who are hypersensitive to antihistamines or to any of the tablet ingredients, and patients who have been treated with MAOIs within the last 14 days

Continued

Side effects

Drowsiness, lassitude, dizziness, dry mouth, blurred vision, headache, gastrointestinal disturbances; IV may cause transient hypotension, CNS stimulation and may be an irritant; inability to concentrate, hepatitis – including jaundice, urinary retention, palpitations, arrhythmias, hypotension, chest tightness, blood disorders including haemolytic anaemia

Allergic reactions: exfoliative dermatitis, photosensitivity, twitching, urticaria, muscle weakness, incoordination, tinnitus, depression, irritability, nightmares

Interactions

Alcohol – potentiates sedative action

Antidepressants – enhance sedative effect – anticholinergic effect intensified with MAOIs

Antidiabetics – depressed thrombocyte count

Antiepileptics – inhibits metabolism of phenytoin

Antihistamines – concomitant therapy NOT recommended

Anxiolytics and hypnotics – enhance the sedative effect

Pharmacodynamic properties

Chlorpheniramine is a potent antihistamine (H_1 antagonist)

Antihistamines diminish or abolish the actions of histamine in the body by competitive reversible blockade of histamine H_1-receptor sites on tissues. Chlorpheniramine also has anticholinergic activity

Prevents release of histamine, prostaglandins and leukotrienes, and has been shown to prevent the migration of inflammatory mediators

The actions of chlorpheniramine include inhibition of histamine on smooth muscle, capillary permeability and hence reduction of oedema and wheal in hypersensitivity reactions such as allergy and anaphylaxis

Fetal risk
No adequate data available in relation to chlorphenira-mine maleate in pregnant women. Use during the third trimester may result in reactions in the newborn or premature neonates. Not to be used during pregnancy unless considered essential by a physician

Breastfeeding
Chlorpheniramine maleate and other antihistamines may inhibit lactation and may be secreted in breast milk. Manufacturers recommend not to be used during lactation

References and Recommended Reading

Baxter, K., 2011. Stockley's Drug Interaction Companion. Pharmaceutical Press, London.

Briggs, G., Freeman, R., Yaffe, S., 2008. Drugs in Pregnancy and Lactation: A Reference Guide to Fetal and Neonatal Risk, eighth ed. Lippincott Williams and Wilkins, Philadelphia.

Bubimschi, C., Weiner, C., 2010. Medication. In: James, D.K., Steer, P.J., Weiner, C.P., Gonik, B. (Eds.), High Risk Pregnancy: Management Options, fourth ed. Elsevier Saunders, London, pp. 579–598.

Chlorphenamine maleate -non-proprietary, see BNF 62, 2011.

Hofmeyr, G.J., Neilson, J.P., Alfreirevic, Z., Crowther, C., Duley, L., Gulmezoglu, M., Gyte, G.M., Hodnett, E.D., 2008. Pregnancy and Childbirth – A Cochrane Pocketbook. Wiley Cochrane Series, London.

Joint Formulary Committee, 2011. British National Formulary (BNF) 62. Pharmaceutical Press, London.

Jordan, S., 2010. Pharmacology for Midwives: The Evidence Base for Safe Practice, second ed. Palgrave Macmillan, Basingstoke.

Koren, G., 2007. Medication Safety in Pregnancy and Breastfeeding: The Evidence Based A–Z Clinician's Pocket Guide. McGraw-Hill, New York.

Nursing and Midwifery Council (NMC), 2011. Changes to Midwives Exemptions 07/2011. Available: http://www.nmc-uk.org/Documents/Circulars/2011Circulars/nmcCircular07-2011-Midwives-Exemptions.pdf. [accessed 28 March 2012].

Nursing and Midwifery Council (NMC), 2011. Midwives Exemptions – Frequently Asked Questions. Available: http://www.nmc-uk.org/Publications-/Circulars/Midwives-exemptions-frequently-asked-questions/ [accessed 28 March 2012].

Rubin, P.C., Ramsey, M., 2007. Prescribing in Pregnancy, fourth ed. BMJ Books/Blackwell Publishing, Oxford.

Schaefer, C., Peters, P.W.J., Miller, R.K. (Eds.), 2007. Drugs During Pregnancy and Lactation: Treatment Options and Risk Assessment, Academic Press/Elsevier, London.

SPC from the eMC, Piriton® tablets, GlaxoSmithKline Consumer Healthcare, updated on the eMC 28/05/2010.

Volans, G., Wiseman, H., 2012. Drugs Handbook 2012–2013, thirtythree ed. Palgrave Macmillan, Basingstoke

Other antihistamines that are used in the relief of allergies, including hay fever, are:

Fexofenadine – non-proprietary, see BNF 62, 2011.

SPC from the eMC, Benadryl® Allergy Relief, McNeil Products Ltd, updated on the eMC 03/04/08.

SPC from the eMC, Clarityn®, Merck Sharp & Dohme Ltd, updated on the eMC 22/02/11.

ALL of the above are not recommended for use in pregnancy, and the risk of embryotoxicity is high with **loratadine** and **fexofenadine**.

11

Antihypertensives

These are substances used to control or modify blood pressure, either by reducing peripheral resistance or blocking α or β adrenoreceptors in the heart, or by reducing the central flow of impulses to the sympathetic nerves and decreasing the release of noradrenaline (norepinephrine) at adrenergic nerve endings.

The student should be aware of:

- the physiology and pathophysiology of blood pressure
- the aetiology, pathophysiology and progression of pregnancy-induced hypertension and pre-eclampsia
- the difference between chronic hypertension (mild, moderate or severe), gestational hypertension, pre-eclampsia, severe pre-eclampsia and eclampsia (NICE, 2010, p5)
- the maternal and fetal sequelae of therapy using these substances
- the local protocols for treatment in cases of eclampsia (see Chapter 25, Emergency drugs, e.g. magnesium sulphate)

NOTE: NICE guideline (CG107, 2010, p18 & p20) lists other medications that may be used during childbearing in some instances: **atenalol, captopril, enalapril** and **metoprolol.** Specific information for these medications should be sought if used for treatments in local NHS Trusts.

BP
Nifedipine

Proprietary
Adalat® (Bayer PLC)
Nifedipine (non-proprietary, see BNF for details)

Group
Calcium channel blocker, hypotensive, vasodilator

Uses/indications
Hypertensive crisis, uncontrolled hypertension
myometrial relaxant – see Chapter 18

Type of drug
POM

Presentation
(Soft) capsules, tablets (modified or prolonged release)

Dosage
Hypertension: 10 mg stat, 10 mg b.d.
Tocolytic: see Chapter 18 for regimen if used as
myometial relaxant

Route of admin
Oral (preferably sublingual during hypertensive crisis)

Contraindications
Continuous use in pregnancy, breastfeeding,
hypersensitivity

Side effects
Headache, flushing, dizziness, oedema, may inhibit
labour
CAUTION: stop treatment if ischaemic pain occurs
within 30–60 min of administration; treatment with
short-acting nifedipine, i.e. during a crisis, can induce an
exaggerated fall in blood pressure and reflex tachycardia, which may cause complications such as cerebrovascular accident/ischaemia or myocardial ischaemia
EXTREME CAUTION when using magnesium sulphate

Interactions
Do not take with grapefruit juice
Antihypertensives – causes severe hypotension and
possible heart failure
Cimetidine – potentiates the hypotensive effect as
metabolism of nifedipine is inhibited

Phenytoin – concomitant administration can reduce the effect of nifedipine – monitor plasma levels of anticonvulsants

Erythromycin – may potentiate nifedipine effects

Insulin – possible impaired glucose tolerance

Pharmacodynamic properties
Selective calcium channel blocker with mostly vascular effects. It is a specific and potent calcium antagonist that relaxes smooth arterial muscle, causing arteries to widen, thereby reducing the resistance in coronary and peripheral circulation. This reduces blood pressure and decreases the heart's overall workload

Fetal risk
Contraindicated in pregnancy before week 20; toxicity and teratogenicity in animals; hypotensive effect can reduce placental flow and cause decrease in fetal oxygenation; may inhibit labour

Breastfeeding
No known adverse side effects (NICE, 2010), but manufacturer advises avoidance

---

BP
Methyldopa

Proprietary
Aldomet® (Aspen)

Methyldopa (Actavis UK Ltd)

Methyldopa (non-proprietary, see BNF for details)

Group
Centrally acting antihypertensive

Uses/indications
Hypertension in pregnancy, hypertensive crisis where immediate effect is not necessary, can be used by asthmatics

Type of drug
POM

Presentation
Tablets

Dosage
Oral: 250 mg b.d. (t.d.s.) max 3 g/day, gradually increased at intervals of 2 days or more

Route of admin
Oral

Contraindications
History of depression, liver disease, phaeochromocytoma, concurrent treatment with MAOIs, porphyria, history of hepatic or renal dysfunction

Side effects
Reduced if under 1 g/day, dry mouth, sedation, depression, fluid retention, haemolytic anaemia, SLE-like syndrome, postural hypotension, gastrointestinal disturbances, dizziness, headache, numbness, hyperprolactinaemia, nightmares, mild psychosis, blood disorders, nasal congestion, nerve and joint pain, hepatic disorders; may interfere with laboratory results – 20% have a positive DCT – advise laboratory of treatment if requiring crossmatch

Interactions
Sympathomimetics, phenothiazines, tricyclic antidepressants and MAOIs – diminish effect
Alcohol – enhances hypotensive effect
Anaesthetics – enhances hypotensive effect ++
Analgesics – NSAIDs enhance hypotensive effect
Antihypertensives – potentiate hypotensive effect
Anxiolytics and hypnotics – enhance hypotensive effect
Corticosteroids – antagonize hypotensive effect
Contraceptives – antagonize hypotensive effect
Iron – possible reduction in the bioavailability of ferrous sulphate or ferrous gluconate if ingested with methyldopa
Salbutamol – use with caution as it can potentiate the hypotensive effect

Pharmacodynamic properties
Methyldopa is metabolized to α-methylnoradrenaline, which lowers arterial pressure (stimulates central inhibitory α-adrenergic receptors), limiting neurotransmission, and/or reduction of plasma renin activity. Withdrawal of the drug is followed by a return of hypertension within 48 h

Fetal risk
Crosses the placental barrier and is present in cord blood; there are theoretical risks of toxicity/teratogenicity including neural development (IQ and links to ADHD)

Breastfeeding
Found in breast milk, and although there are no obvious effects the manufacturer advises that lactating mothers be warned of its presence and possible risk, but does not advise avoidance

BP
Hydralazine hydrochloride

Proprietary
Apresoline® 20 mg ampoules (Sovereign Medical)
Apresoline® 25 mg tablets (Amdipharm PLC)
Hydralazine (non-proprietary, see BNF for details)

Group
Antihypertensive – vasodilator

Uses/indications
Raised diastolic blood pressure used concomitantly with other therapies, e.g. beta-blockers or during a hypertensive crisis

Type of drug
POM

Presentation
Tablets, injection, powder for reconstitution

Continued

Dosage
Oral: 25–50 mg b.d.
Slow IV injection: 5–10 mg over 20 min, repeated after
20–30 min – diluted with sodium chloride 0.9%
IV infusion: 200–300 mcg/min
Maintenance: 5–150 mcg/min

Route of admin
Oral, IV injection or infusion

Contraindications
Systemic lupus erythematosus (SLE), tachycardia, hepatic,
renal or cardiac dysfunction, or cerebrovascular accident

Side effects
Nausea, postural hypotension, tachycardia, palpitations,
flushing, fluid retention, after prolonged or high-dose
therapy SLE-like syndrome, headache, dizziness, joint,
muscle and nerve pain, nasal congestion, blood
disorders, liver and renal disorders

Interactions
Alcohol – enhances hypotensive effect
Anaesthetics – enhances hypotensive effect
Analgesics – NSAIDs enhance hypotensive effect
Antihypertensives – enhance hypotensive effect
Anxiolytics and hypnotics – enhance the hypotensive
effects
Contraceptives – combined oral contraceptives
antagonize the hypotensive effect

Pharmacodynamic properties
Acts on the smooth muscle tissue surrounding the
arteries, causing them to relax and hence the blood
pressure to fall

Fetal risk
Toxicity in animals, therefore considered a teratogen,
although there are no reported links to congenital
defects in humans. Avoid before the third trimester, but
there are no reports of serious harm

Breastfeeding
No known adverse side effects (NICE, 2010) and thus considered safe, but infant requires monitoring

---

BP
Labetalol hydrochloride

Proprietary
Trandate® (UCB Pharma Ltd)
Labetalol (non-proprietary, see BNF for details),

Group
Antihypertensive – α and β adrenoreceptor blocker

Uses/indications
Hypertension in pregnancy, hypertensive crisis

Type of drug
POM

Presentation
Tablets, ampoules

Dosage
Oral: initial dose 100 mg b.d. increased at weekly intervals by 100 mg b.d., to 200 mg b.d.
In the second and third trimesters further dose titration to t.d.s., ranging from 100 to 400 mg t.d.s.; can be increased up to 800 mg in three to four evenly divided doses/day (max 2.4 g daily)
IV injection: 50 mg over 1 min repeated after 5 min (max 200 mg)
IV infusion: 20 mg/h doubled after 30 min (max 160 mg/h)

Route of admin
Oral, IV injection or infusion

Contraindications
Asthma, chronic obstructive airway disease, wheezing, phaeochromocytoma, bradycardia, sensitivity to labetalol, heart block, Raynaud's disease, use with caution in patients with psoriasis

Continued

Side effects
Postural hypotension – particularly 3 h after IV administration, tiredness, weakness, epigastric pain, difficulty with micturition, scalp tingling, tremor in pregnant patients

Interactions
Alcohol – enhances hypotensives effect as delays metabolism of labetalol

Anaesthetics – enhance hypotensive effect

Analgesics – NSAIDs enhance hypotensive effects

Antacids – cimetidine inhibits the metabolism and therefore increases the plasma concentration of labetalol

Antidepressants – tricyclics cause tremor; MAOIs not recommended

Antidiabetics – enhanced hypoglycaemic effects and masks warning signs such as tremor

Antihistamines – increased risk of ventricular arrhythmia with terfenadine

Antihypertensives – concomitant use may cause severe hypotension

Anxiolytics and hypnotics – enhance the hypotensive effect

Corticosteroids – antagonize the hypotensive effect

Ergometrine – increases peripheral vasoconstriction

Contraceptives – combined oral contraceptives antagonize the hypotensive effect

Pharmacodynamic properties
Works by blocking peripheral arteriolar α receptors and this reduces peripheral resistance. A concurrent β-blockade protects the heart from any reflux effects. Cardiac output is not significantly reduced at rest or after moderate exercise, i.e. the increase in systolic pressure during exercise is reduced and the diastolic pressure remains essentially normal

Fetal risk
Manufacturer advise labetalol should be used only in the first trimester if benefit outweighs risk; caution in use – β-blockers reduce placental perfusion, leading to a risk of intrauterine death, premature delivery, fetal growth deficiency, and increased risk of neonatal hypoglycaemia and bradycardia, respiratory depression and neonatal jaundice. The risk is greater in severe hypertension and with multiple therapy, although these effects may be due to the disease itself and not the therapy. These symptoms can develop 1–2 days after delivery

Breastfeeding
Excreted in breast milk; although manufacturers recommend avoidance, no known adverse side effects (NICE, 2010)

References and Recommended Reading

Baxter, K., 2011. Stockley's Drug Interaction Companion. Pharmaceutical Press, London.

Bewley, C., 2011. Hypertensive disorders of pregnancy. In: Macdonald, S., Magill-Cuerden, J. (Eds.), Mayes' Midwifery, fourteenth ed. Baillière Tindall/Elsevier, Edinburgh, pp. 787–798.

Briggs, G., Freeman, R., Yaffe, S., 2008. Drugs in Pregnancy and Lactation: A Reference Guide to Fetal and Neonatal Risk, eighth ed. Lippincott Williams and Wilkins, Philadelphia.

Bubimschi, C., Weiner, C., 2010. Medication. In: James, D.K., Steer, P.J., Weiner, C.P., Gonik, B. (Eds.), High Risk Pregnancy: Management Options, fourth ed. Elsevier Saunders, London, pp. 579–598.

Centre for Maternal and Child Enquiries 2011. Saving Mothers' Lives, Reviewing Maternal Deaths to Make Motherhood Safer: 2006–2008. The 8th Report of the Confidential Enquiries into Maternal Deaths in the United Kingdom. Available http://www.oaa-anaes.ac.uk/assets/_managed/editor/File/Reports/2006-2008%20CEMD.pdf [accessed 2 March 2012].

Dekker, G., 2010. Hypertension. In: James, D.K., Steer, P.J., Weiner, C.P., Gonik, B. (Eds.), High Risk Pregnancy: Management Options, fourth ed. Elsevier Saunders, London, pp. 599–626.

Joint Formulary Committee, 2011. British National Formulary (BNF) 62. Pharmaceutical Press, London.

Jordan, S. (Ed.), 2010. Pharmacology for Midwives: The Evidence Base for Safe Practice, second ed. Palgrave Macmillan, Basingstoke.

Koren, G., 2007. Medication Safety in Pregnancy and Breastfeeding: The Evidence Based A–Z Clinician's Pocket Guide. McGraw-Hill, New York.

National Institute of Clinical Excellence (NICE), 2010. CG107 Hypertension in Pregnancy. NICE, London.

Rubin, P.C., Ramsey, M., 2007. Prescribing in Pregnancy, fourth ed. BMJ Books/Blackwell Publishing, Oxford.

Schaefer, C., Peters, P.W.J., Miller, R.K. (Eds.), 2007. Drugs During Pregnancy and Lactation: Treatment Options and Risk Assessment, Academic Press/Elsevier, London.

SPC from the eMC, Adalat®, Bayer PLC, updated on the eMC 22/9/11.

SPC from the eMC, Aldomet® 250 mg and 500 mg tablets, Aspen, updated on the eMC 13/7/11.

SPC from the eMC, Apresoline® 20 mg ampoules, Sovereign Medical, updated on the eMC 13/4/10.

SPC from the eMC, Apresoline® 25 mg tablets, Amdipharm UK Ltd, updated on the eMC 16/2/11.

SPC from the eMC, Methyldopa 125 mg, 250 mg, 500 mg tablets, Actavis UK Ltd, updated on the eMC 17/1/11.

Trandate® 50 mg, 100 mg, 200 mg and 400 mg tablets (Labetalol hydrochloride), UCB Pharma Ltd, updated in BNF 62, 2011.

Trandate® 5 mg/mL injection, UCB Pharma Ltd, updated in BNF 62, 2011.

12

Antiseptics

These substances are also known as disinfectants, bacteriostats, bactericides and germicides. They inhibit the growth of, or kill, microorganisms. Antiseptics are usually applied to the body or as disinfectants to equipment, etc. Skin cleansers are also included in this chapter.

The student should be aware of:

■ the difference between antiseptics and antibiotics
■ local Trust guidance for infection control.

BP
Surgical alcohol (Isopropyl alcohol)

Proprietary
Sterets® (Mölnlycke Health Care)

Group
Alcohol-based cleanser

Uses/indications
Preparation of the skin prior to injection

Type of drug
GSL

Presentation
Injection swabs

Dosage
N/A

Route of admin
Topical

Continued

Contraindications
Broken skin, patients with burns, prior to using diathermy

Side effects
Flammable, skin irritation

Interactions
N/A

Pharmacodynamic properties
70% isopropyl alcohol has disinfectant properties and, when used in combination with chlorhexidine, has antimicrobial qualities; therefore it is used to clean the skin and reduce the bacteriological count prior to injection or surgery

Fetal risk
N/A

Breastfeeding
N/A

BP
Sodium chloride

Proprietary
Sodium chloride (Goldshield Group UK Ltd)
(non-proprietary, see BNF for details)

Group
Saline skin cleanser

Uses/indications
Cleansing of skin and wounds

Presentation
Sterile solution in 2 mL, 5 mL and 10 mL hermetically sealed translucent plastic ampoules

Dosage
N/A

Route of admin
Topical

Contraindications
N/A

Side effects
N/A

Interactions
N/A

Fetal risk
N/A

Breastfeeding
N/A

BP
Povidone–Iodine

Proprietary
Betadine® Surgical Scrub (Mölnlycke Health Care)
Betadine® dry-powder spray (Mölnlycke Health Care)
Videne® (Ecolab)

Group
Antiseptic – iodine compounds

Uses/indications
Skin disinfection, preoperative and postoperative, caution with diathermy

Presentation
Prepared solutions, powders

Dosage
N/A

Route of admin
Topical

Contraindications
Iodine sensitivity, renal impairment, regular use in patients or users with thyroid disorders

Side effects
Sensitivity

Continued

Interactions
N/A

Pharmacodynamic properties
The povidone–iodine slowly liberates iodine on contact with the skin and mucous membranes, and acts as a microbicide, effectively 'suffocating' the microbe by displacing its oxygen supply and altering the stability of the microbial cell membrane

Fetal risk
Avoid regular use in pregnancy and lactation, as iodine compounds cross the placenta – may affect fetal thyroid function in second and third trimesters

Breastfeeding
Iodine compounds are excreted in breast milk, and although no adverse effects have been reported it should be considered hazardous and the possible benefits should be weighed against the risks of thyroid dysfunction and maldevelopment; avoid use on very low-birthweight babies

---

BP
Chlorhexidine gluconate

Proprietary
Hibiscrub® (Mölnlycke Health Care); Hibisol® (Mölnlycke Health Care); Hibitane® Obstetric cream (Centrapharm); Hydrex® (Ecolab)
(non-proprietary, see BNF for details)

Group
Antiseptic – chlorhexidine salts, phenyl derivative

Uses/indications
Skin preparation prior to surgery, cleansing of perineum and vulva, lubrication of the midwife's hands (as Hibitane® Obstetric cream – chlorhexidine gluconate solution 5% in water as lubricant)

Presentation
Prepared solutions of varying concentrations

Dosage
N/A

Route of admin
Topical

Contraindications
Hypersensitivity, avoid contact with the eyes, brain meninges and middle ear; not suitable before diathermy

Side effects
Sensitivity

Interactions
N/A

Pharmacodynamic properties
Wide range of antimicrobial activities against Gram-positive and Gram-negative vegetative bacteria, dermatological fungi and lipophilic viruses. It is inactive against bacterial spores except at raised temperatures. Its cationic nature means that it binds strongly to skin, mucosa and other tissues, and is very poorly absorbed; therefore there are no detectable levels after oral or skin contact

Fetal risk
N/A

Breastfeeding
Considered safe (as used as a handwash)

BP
Chlorhexidine gluconate and Cetrimide solution

Proprietary
Savlon® (Novartis Consumer Health)

Group
Antiseptic – phenyl derivative

Uses/indications
General-purpose antiseptic, disinfectant and detergent

Type of drug
GSL

Presentation
Liquid – chlorhexidine 1.5% : cetrimide 15%

Dosage
As instructed

Route of admin
Topical – diluted for external use only

Contraindications
Sensitivity

Side effects
Contamination by *Pseudomonas aeruginosa* – store as
sterile solutions in screwtop bottles; keep out of eyes
and ears

Interactions
N/A

Fetal risk
N/A

Breastfeeding
N/A

References and Recommended Reading

Betadine® 2.5% dry powder spray, Mölnlycke Health Care, updated in
the BNF 62, 2011.

Briggs, G., Freeman, R., Yaffe, S., 2008. Drugs in Pregnancy and
Lactation: A Reference Guide to Fetal and Neonatal Risk, eighth ed.
Lippincott Williams and Wilkins, Philadelphia.

Joint Formulary Committee, 2011. British National Formulary (BNF) 62.
Pharmaceutical Press, London.

Rubin, P.C., Ramsey, M., 2007. Prescribing in Pregnancy, fourth ed.
BMJ Books/Blackwell Publishing, Oxford.

Schaefer, C., Peters, P.W.J., Miller, R.K. (Eds.), 2007. Drugs During
Pregnancy and Lactation: Treatment Options and Risk Assessment,
Academic Press/Elsevier, London.

SPC from the eMC, Betadine® Surgical Scrub, Mölnlycke Health Care,
updated on the eMC 20/10/06.

SPC from the eMC, Hibiscrub® SSL, Mölnlycke Health Care, updated
on the eMC 20/10/06.

SPC from the eMC, Hibitane® Obstetric Cream, Centrapharm, updated in the BNF 62 2011.

SPC from the eMC, Savlon®, Novartis Consumer Health, updated on the eMC 14/1/09.

SPC from the eMC, Sodium Chloride 0.9% w/v solution for injection, Goldshield Group Ltd, updated on the eMC 17/8/10.

SPC from the eMC, Sterets®, Mölnlycke Health Care, updated on the eMC 20/9/06.

13

Anxiolytics and Hypnotics

These are used to lessen tension and excitement and to induce sleep. They may be prescribed for anxious patients or those unable to sleep in the antenatal period during hospitalization.

The student should be aware of:

- the effects that tension has in exacerbating certain conditions
- the addictive qualities of such preparations.

| **BP** |
| Temazepam |
| **Proprietary**
Temazepam (Sandoz Ltd), 10 mg and 20 mg
(Non-proprietary, see BNF for details) |
| **Group**
Hypnotic – benzodiazepine |
| **Uses/indications**
Insomnia (short-term use) |
| **Type of drug**
POM |
| **Presentation**
Tablets (white) |
| **Dosage**
10–20 mg nocte |

Route of admin
Oral

Contraindications
Any history of drug/alcohol abuse, respiratory disease, myasthenia gravis, marked personality disorders, hypersensitivity to this or benzodiazepines, renal/hepatic disorder, sleep apnoea, muscle weakness

Side effects
Drowsiness, lightheadedness, reduced alertness, confusion, fatigue, muscle weakness, numbed emotion, headache, ataxia, double vision

Interactions
Alcohol, analgesics, anaesthetics, antiepileptics, antihistamines
Antihypertensives – all enhance the sedative effect
Antihistamines – concomitant administration with diphenhydramine can cause intrauterine or early neonatal death

Pharmacodynamic properties
A hypnotic/sedative/anxiolytic results in anxiolysis, muscle relaxation, CNS sedation, possibly acting on GABA receptors to potentiate GABA effects

Fetal risk
Drowsiness; with large doses hypotonia; during last phase of pregnancy or during labour – depression of neonatal respiration, hypothermia and withdrawal symptoms

Breastfeeding
Considered moderately safe but avoid repeated doses – can lead to lethargy and weight loss in the infant

References and Recommended Reading

Baxter, K., 2011. Stockley's Drug Interaction Companion. Pharmaceutical Press, London.

Briggs, G., Freeman, R., Yaffe, S., 2008. Drugs in Pregnancy and Lactation: A Reference Guide to Fetal and Neonatal Risk, eighth ed. Lippincott Williams and Wilkins, Philadelphia.

Bubimschi, C., Weiner, C., 2010. Medication. In: James, D.K., Steer, P.J., Weiner, C.P., Gonik, B. (Eds.), High Risk Pregnancy: Management Options, fourth ed. Elsevier Saunders, London, pp. 579–598.

Joint Formulary Committee, 2011. British National Formulary (BNF) 62. Pharmaceutical Press, London.

Jordan, S., 2010. Pharmacology for Midwives: The Evidence Base for Safe Practice, second ed. Palgrave Macmillan, Basingstoke.

Koren, G., 2007. Medication Safety in Pregnancy and Breastfeeding: The Evidence Based A–Z Clinician's Pocket Guide. McGraw-Hill, New York.

Rubin, P.C., Ramsey, M., 2007. Prescribing in Pregnancy, fourth ed. BMJ Books/Blackwell Publishing, Oxford.

Schaefer, C., Peters, P.W.J., Miller, R.K. (Eds.), 2007. Drugs During Pregnancy and Lactation: Treatment Options and Risk Assessment, Academic Press/Elsevier, London.

SPC from the eMC, Temazepam 10 mg and 20 mg, Sandoz Limited, updated on the eMC 21/12/09.

Volans, G., Wiseman, H., 2012. Drugs Handbook 2012–2013, thirtythird ed. Palgrave Macmillan, Basingstoke.

14

Contraceptives

This is a general term to describe an agent used to prevent conception.

As part of their sphere of practice, midwives have a duty to offer family planning advice (Nursing and Midwifery Council (NMC), 2004; NICE, 2006; Article 42 of the European Union Standards for Nursing and Midwifery, 2009).

The student should be aware of:

- the availability of contraception (hormonal, intrauterine devices, barrier methods, spermicidal and emergency contraception)
- the importance of family planning
- the process of contraception with a view to usage of emergency contraception
- the appropriateness of the contraceptive prescribed
- the importance of counselling – advice on bleeding, missed pills, diarrhoea and vomiting, antibiotic administration, and cessation of oral contraception prior to surgery.

BP
Combined oestrogen–progestogen oral contraceptive (COC)

Proprietary
Marvelon® (Merck Sharp & Dohme Ltd), Yasmin® (Bayer PLC), Femodene® (Bayer PLC), Microgynon 30® ED, (Bayer PLC), Ovranette® (Pfizer Ltd), Loestrin 20® and Loestrin 30® (Galen Ltd), Millinette® 20/75 (Consilient Health Ltd)

Group
Contraceptive – hormonal

Continued

Uses/indications
Contraception, menstrual symptoms

Type of drug
POM

Presentation
Tablets in packs for 1 month, with days numbered

Dosage
Usually 1 tablet/day, but refer to pack for instructions
Postpartum (not breastfeeding) – commence at
3 weeks' postpartum – there is an increased risk of DVT
if commenced earlier – patient must be fully ambulant,
with no puerperal complications, and be counselled for
the risk of DVT

Breastfeeding – not recommended until weaning or at
least 6 months if unable to obtain other contraception

Miscarriage or abortion – commence on same day if
possible

Route of admin
Oral

Contraindications
Pregnancy, migraine, liver disease including cholestatic
jaundice, history of pruritus in pregnancy, breastfeeding, prothrombotic coagulation disorders, previous
history or strong familial history of DVT, undiagnosed
vaginal bleeding, breast or genital tract carcinoma
CAUTION: arterial disease, smoking, hypertension,
obesity, diabetes mellitus with retinopathy and
nephropathy, ischaemic heart disease, varicosities,
depression, inflammatory bowel disease, Rotor
syndrome, Dubin–Johnson syndrome, sickle cell
anaemia, history of herpes gestationis, disorders of lipid
metabolism
Stop prior to major surgery or surgery to the legs, or
with long-term immobilization – do not stop for minor
surgery with short anaesthetic duration, e.g. laparos-
copy or tooth extraction

Side effects
Nausea, vomiting, headache, breast tenderness, changes in body weight, libido changes, DVT, intracycle bleeding, amenorrhoea, decreased menstrual bleeding, depression, impaired liver function

Interactions
Antibiotics – broad spectrum – reduce effect
Anticoagulants – antagonizes the effect of warfarin
Antidepressants – tricyclics – antagonizes the antidepressant effects but increases the side effects because of the increased plasma concentration of tricyclics
Antidiabetics – antagonism of the hypoglycaemic effect
Antiepileptics – carbamazepine, phenobarbital and phenytoin accelerate metabolism and reduce contraceptive effect
Antihypertensives – antagonize hypotensive effect

Pharmacodynamic properties
The combination of these preparations acts to inhibit ovulation by suppressing the mid-cycle surge of luteinizing hormone, thickening the cervical mucus as a barrier to sperm, and rendering the endometrium unresponsive to implantation

Fetal risk
Evidence suggests no harmful effects to fetus, although there is teratogenicity in animals (US studies have found a small risk of 0.07% of all pregnancies exposed to the oral contraceptive pill)

Breastfeeding
Suppressed lactation; contraindicated until at least 6 months after birth

BP
Progestogen-only pill (POP)

Proprietary
Cerazette® (Merck Sharp & Dohme Ltd), Femulen® (Pharmcia Ltd), Micronor® (Janssen Cilag Ltd), Norgeston® (Bayer PLC), Noriday® (Pfizer Ltd)

Group
Contraceptive – hormonal

Uses/indications
Contraception, alternative to oestrogens – higher failure rate, suitable in smokers, hypertension, valvular heart disease, diabetes mellitus, migraine, predisposition to or history of thrombosis or venous thrombosis

Type of drug
POM

Presentation
Tablets in cyclical packs

Dosage
Usually 1 tablet/day, but refer to pack instructions – must be taken at the same time each day
postpartum – commence after 3 weeks – breakthrough bleeding if earlier – women should also be aware of the increased risk of thromboembolic disorders

Route of admin
Oral

Contraindications
Pregnancy, undiagnosed vaginal bleeding, severe arterial disease, existing thrombophlebitis or thrombo-embolic disorders, cerebrovascular disease, porphyria, heart disease including myocardial infarction, malab-sorption syndromes, liver disease, sex steroid-dependent cancers, past ectopic pregnancy, functional ovarian cysts, cholestatic jaundice, pruritus of pregnancy, Dubin–Johnson syndrome, Rotor syndrome, history of herpes gestationis, disorders of lipid metabolism

Side effects
Menstrual irregularities, nausea, vomiting, menstrual symptoms, weight change, depression, dizziness, loss of libido, headaches, chloasma

Interactions
Antibiotics – rifamycins – increase metabolism and therefore reduce effect
Anticoagulants – antagonize effect of warfarin
Antidiabetics – antagonize the hypoglycaemic effects
Antiepileptics – reduce contraceptive effect
St John's wort – can lead to potential loss of contraceptive effect

Pharmacodynamic properties
POPs have a progestational effect on the endometrium and cervical mucus that discourages implantation and decreases corpus luteum function

Fetal risk
High doses may be teratogenic in the first trimester (US studies have found a 0.07 % risk) and cause masculinization of the fetus, although only with very high progestogen doses

Breastfeeding
Not contraindicated, but not before 3 weeks' postpartum. Manufacturer advises avoidance, as small amounts of active ingredients are excreted in breast milk and the effects on the infant are unknown

BP
Etonogestrel

Proprietary
Implanon® (Merck Sharp & Dohme Ltd)

Group
Parenteral progestogen-only contraceptive

Continued

Uses/indications
Contraception effective for up to 3 years – rapidly reversible on removal

Type of drug
POM

Presentation
Non-biodegradable white to off-white flexible rod

Dosage
68 mg etonogestrel in each rod with no previous hormonal contraception: one implant in the first 5 days of the cycle
Parturition/abortion in second trimester: 1 implant 21–28 days after delivery or abortion

Route of admin
Subdermal

Contraindications
As for progestogen-only pill

Side effects
Aching, pain at site, tiredness, acne, alopecia, headache, dizziness, depression, mood swings, libido changes, gastrointestinal disturbances, weight changes, menstrual symptoms, occasional hypertension, vaginal infection, acne, increased risk of DVT

Interactions
As for progestogen-only pill

Pharmacodynamic properties
A progestogen that inhibits progesterone receptors in target organs. Primarily it works to inhibit ovulation, and also to thicken the cervical mucus, making it hostile to spermatozoa

Fetal risk
As for progestogen-only pill

Breastfeeding
As for progestogen-only pill

BP
Medroxyprogesterone acetate

Proprietary
Depo-Provera® (Pharmacia Ltd)

Group
Parenteral progesterone-only contraceptive

Uses/indications
Depo-Provera is a long-term contraceptive agent
suitable for use in women who have been appropriately
counselled concerning the likelihood of menstrual
disturbance and the potential for a delay in return to
full fertility. Depo-Provera may also be used for
short-term contraception in the following
circumstances:

- for partners of men undergoing vasectomy, for
  protection until the vasectomy becomes effective
- in women who are being immunized against rubella,
  to prevent pregnancy during the period of activity of
  the virus
- in women awaiting sterilization

Type of drug
POM

Presentation
Aqueous suspension in vials

Dosage
150 mg in first 5 days of menstrual cycle or within 5 days
of parturition; repeat in 12 weeks

Route of admin
IM

Contraindications
As for progestogen-only preparations

Continued

Side effects
Common side effects: menstrual irregularities (bleeding and/or amenorrhoea), weight changes, headache, nervousness, abdominal pain or discomfort, dizziness, asthenia (weakness or fatigue)
Adverse events reported by 1–5%: decreased libido or anorgasmia, backache, leg cramps, depression, nausea, insomnia, leucorrhoea, acne, vaginitis, pelvic pain, breast pain, no hair growth or alopecia, bloating, rash, oedema, hot flushes

Interactions
As for progestogen-only preparations

Pharmacodynamic properties
Exerts an antiandrogenic and antigonadotrophic effect that inhibits ovulation and endometrial preparation for pregnancy

Fetal risk
Possible increase in low birthweight that is associated with increased risk of neonatal death – although the attributable risk is low as pregnancies are uncommon. Those exposed show no adverse effects

Breastfeeding
Secreted into breast milk but no evidence of harmful effects; may be advised to withhold for the first 6 weeks postnatally if breastfeeding

---

BP
Norethisterone enanthate

Proprietary
Noristerat® (Bayer PLC)

Group
Parenteral progestogen-only contraceptive

Uses/indications
Short-term or interim contraception, 8 weeks' duration

Type of drug
POM

Presentation
Oily preparation in ampoules

Dosage
Deep IM: 200 mg in first 5 days of cycle or immediately after parturition; repeat in 8 weeks

Route of admin
Deep IM

Contraindications
As for progestogen-only preparations

Side effects
As for progestogen-only preparations

Interactions
As for progestogen-only preparations

Fetal risk
As for progestogen-only preparations

Breastfeeding
Withhold when neonate has severe jaundice requiring medical treatment; may also suppress lactation in high doses and alter composition of breast milk, therefore use the lowest effective dose

---

BP
Levonorgestrel

Proprietary
Levonell® One Step (Bayer PLC)

Group
Emergency contraception

Uses/indications
Emergency contraception within 72 h (3 days) of unprotected sexual intercourse or failure of a contraceptive method

Type of drug
POM (GSL over 16 years of age by pharmacists only)

Continued

Presentation
Tablets

Dosage
1 tablet (1500 mcg levonorgestrel) should be taken as
soon as possible, preferably within 12 h and no later
than 72 h after unprotected intercourse

Route of admin
Oral

Contraindications
Pregnancy, porphyria, overdue menstrual bleeding or
unprotected intercourse more than 72 h previously,
bowel disease, liver disease, history of ectopic
pregnancy, salpingitis, and the use of some other
medications

Side effects
Nausea, abdominal pain, vomiting, headache, fatigue,
breast discomfort

Interactions
The metabolism of levonorgestrel is enhanced by
concomitant use of liver enzyme inducers
Possible drugs suspected of reducing the efficacy of
levonorgestrel-containing medication include barbiturates (including primidone), phenytoin, carbamazepine,
herbal medicines containing *Hypericum perforatum*
(St John's wort), rifampicin, ritonavir, rifabutin,
griseofulvin. Women taking such drugs should be
referred to their doctor for advice

Pharmacodynamic properties
Inhibits ovulation if taken in the preovulatory stage, and
also causes endometrial changes that discourage
implantation. However, once implantation has occurred
it is no longer an effective contraceptive. It is effective in
up to 84% when given within 72 h of intercourse
(3 days)

Fetal risk

Abortifacient, but pregnancy may continue; monitor for signs of ectopic pregnancy. In theory, because there is no organogenesis at 72 h there should be no teratogenicity

Breastfeeding

Exposure of the infant is reduced if the mother avoids nursing post medication

References and Recommended Reading

Baxter, K., 2011. Stockley's Drug Interaction Companion. Pharmaceutical Press, London.

Briggs, G., Freeman, R., Yaffe, S., 2008. Drugs in Pregnancy and Lactation: A Reference Guide to Fetal and Neonatal Risk, eighth ed. Lippincott Williams and Wilkins, Philadelphia.

Bubimschi, C., Weiner, C., 2010. Medication. In: James, D.K., Steer, P.J., Weiner, C.P., Gonik, B. (Eds.), High Risk Pregnancy: Management Options, fourth ed. Elsevier Saunders, London, pp. 579–598.

Hofmeyr, G.J., Neilson, J.P., Alfreirevic, Z., Crowther, C., Duley, L., Gulmezoglu, M., Gyte, G.M., Hodnett, E.D., 2008. Pregnancy and Childbirth – A Cochrane Pocketbook. Wiley Cochrane Series, London.

Joint Formulary Committee, 2011. British National Formulary (BNF) 62. Pharmaceutical Press, London.

Jordan, S. (Ed.), 2010. Pharmacology for Midwives: The Evidence Base for Safe Practice, second ed. Palgrave Macmillan, Basingstoke.

Koren, G., 2007. Medication Safety in Pregnancy and Breastfeeding: The Evidence Based A–Z Clinician's Pocket Guide. McGraw-Hill, New York.

National Institute for Health and Clinical Excellence (NICE), 2006. CG37 Postnatal Care. NICE, London.

Nursing and Midwifery Council (NMC), 2004. Midwives Rules and Standards. NMC, London.

Rubin, P.C., Ramsey, M., 2007. Prescribing in Pregnancy, fourth ed. BMJ Books/Blackwell Publishing, Oxford.

Schaefer, C., Peters, P.W.J., Miller, R.K. (Eds.), 2007. Drugs During Pregnancy and Lactation: Treatment Options and Risk Assessment, Academic Press/Elsevier, London.

SPC from the eMC, Cerazette®, Merck Sharp & Dohme, updated on the eMC 19/06/08.

SPC from the eMC, Depo-Provera®, Pharmacia Ltd, updated on the eMC 25/01/12.

SPC from the eMC, ellaOne®, HRA Pharma UK, updated on the eMC 20/12/11.

SPC from the eMC, Femodene® ED, Bayer PLC, updated on the eMC 13/05/11.

SPC from the eMC, Femulen®, Pharmacia Ltd, updated on the eMC 04/03/08.

SPC from the eMC, Gygel®, Marlborough Pharmaceuticals Ltd, updated on the eMC 08/01/11.

SPC from the eMC, Implanon®, Merck Sharp & Dohme Ltd, updated on the eMC 10/10/09.

SPC from the eMC, Levonell®, One Step, Bayer PLC, updated on the eMC 11/11/10.

PIL from the eMC, Loestrin 20® and Loestrin 30®, Galen Ltd, updated on the eMC 27/03/12.

SPC from the eMC, Marvelon®, Merck Sharp & Dohme Ltd, updated on the eMC 06/06/11.

SPC from the eMC, Microgynon 30® ED, Bayer PLC, updated on the eMC 28/06/11.

SPC from the eMC, Micronor®, Janssen Cilag Ltd, updated on the eMC 29/02/12.

PIL from the eMC, Millinette® 20/75, Consilient Health Ltd, updated on the eMC 02/07/10.

SPC from the eMC, Mirena®, Bayer PLC, updated on the eMC 05/01/12.

SPC from the eMC, Nexplanon®, Merck Sharp & Dohme Ltd, updated on the eMC 20/10/10.

SPC from the eMC, Norgeston®, Bayer PLC, updated on the eMC 07/03/11.

SPC from the eMC, Noriday®, Pfizer Ltd, updated on the eMC 16/08/10.

SPC from the eMC, Noristerat®, Bayer PLC, updated on the eMC 18/06/09.

SPC from the eMC, Ovranette®, Pfizer Ltd, updated on the eMC 31/08/11.

SPC from the eMC, Yasmin®, Bayer PLC, updated on the eMC 07/10/11.

Towse, R., 2011. Fertility and its control. In: Macdonald, S., Magill-Cuerden, J. (Eds.), Mayes' Midwifery, fourteenth ed. Baillière Tindall/Elsevier, Edinburgh, pp. 327–338.

Volans, G., Wiseman, H., 2012. Drugs Handbook 2012–2013, thirtythird ed. Palgrave Macmillan, Basingstoke.

World Health Organization, 2009. European Union Standard for Nursing and Midwifery: Information for Accession Countries. Available http://www.euro.who.int/__data/assets/pdf_file/0005/102200/E92852.pdf [accessed 14 May 2012].

15

Emergency Drugs

This chapter includes some of the drugs used in emergencies such as cardiac arrest, anaphylaxis and eclampsia (see Chapters 16 and 17 for drugs for haemorrhage).

Each student should quickly become familiar with the local protocols and policies that cover such emergencies and seek adequate training in resuscitation techniques.

Drugs Used in the Treatment of Cardiac Arrest

Cardiac arrest may be associated with ventricular fibrillation, pulseless ventricular tachycardia, asystole and pulseless electrical activity (electromechanical dissociation).

NB: Atropine is no longer recommended in the treatment of asystole or pulseless electrical activity.

BP
Adrenaline (epinephrine)

Proprietary
Cardiac arrest
Adrenaline (Epinephrine) 1:10000 Sterile Solution Minijet® (International Medication Systems (UK) Ltd)
Anaphylaxis
Adrenaline (Epinephrine) Injection BP 1 in 1000 (Hameln Pharmaceuticals Ltd)

Group
Cardiopulmonary resuscitation, allergic emergencies

Uses/indications
Asystolic cardiac arrest in conjunction with calcium chloride and defibrillation. Increases cardiac output and force of contractility by producing generalized vasoconstriction by acting on vascular smooth muscle **anaphylactic shock** or severe allergic reactions

Type of drug
POM

Presentation
Minijet, ampoules, auto-injector, prefilled pen, prefilled syringe

Dosage
Cardiac arrest:

Adrenaline (Epinephrine) 1 : 10 000:
- 10 mL (1 mg) by IV injection repeated every 2–3 min as necessary
- 1–10 mL (0.1–1 mg) direct into atrium of heart

Sodium Chloride 0.9% injection: 20 mL peripherally must be administered following adrenaline to aid entry into the central circulation (BNF 62, 2011)

Anaphylactic shock:

Adrenaline Injection BP 1/1000: 500 mcq (0.5 mL adrenaline 1/1000). May be repeated several times at 5-min intervals according to blood pressure, pulse and respiratory function

Route of admin
Cardiac arrest: Adrenaline (Ephedrine) 1 : 10 000 – IV (if administered via a central line must not interrupt CPR), intracardiac injection or intraosseous route

Anaphylaxis: Adrenaline Injection BP 1/1000 – S.C./ IM/IV (UK Resuscitation Council, 2010, recommends IM)

Continued

NB: the needle used needs to be long enough to ensure that adrenaline is injected into the muscle; IV use restricted to specialists

Contraindications
Cardiac arrest: Adrenaline (Epinephrine) 1 : 10 000
Contraindications are relative as this product is intended for use in life-threatening emergencies
other than in the emergency situation, the following contraindications should be considered. hyperthyroidism, hypertension, ischaemic heart disease, diabetes mellitus and closed-angle glaucoma
Anaphylaxis: Adrenaline Injection BP 1/1000
Use during labour
With local anaesthesia of peripheral structures including digits, ear lobe
In the presence of ventricular fibrillation, cardiac dilatation, coronary insufficiency, organic brain disease or atherosclerosis, except in emergencies where the potential benefit clearly outweighs the risk
If the solution is discoloured

Side effects
Ventricular fibrillation may occur and severe hypertension may lead to cerebral haemorrhage and pulmonary oedema
Symptomatic adverse effects are anxiety, dyspnoea, restlessness, palpitations, tachycardia, anginal pain, tremor, weakness, dizziness, headache and cold extremities
Biochemical effects include inhibition of insulin secretion, stimulation of growth hormone secretion, hyperglycaemia (even with low doses), gluconeogenesis, glycolysis, lipolysis and ketogenesis

Interactions
The effects of adrenaline may be potentiated by **tricyclic antidepressants**

Volatile **liquid anaesthetics** such as halothane increase the risk of adrenaline-induced ventricular arrhythmias and acute pulmonary oedema if hypoxia is present

Severe hypertension and bradycardia may occur with non-selective **beta-blocking drugs** such as propranolol

Propranolol also inhibits the bronchodilator effect of adrenaline

Risk of cardiac arrhythmias is higher when adrenaline is given to patients receiving **digoxin** or **quinidine**

Risk of hypertensive crisis with **MAOIs**

Adrenaline-induced hyperglycaemia may lead to loss of blood-sugar control in diabetic patients treated with **hypoglycaemic agents**

The vasoconstrictor and pressor effects of adrenaline, mediated by its α-adrenergic action, may be enhanced by concomitant administration of drugs with similar effects, such as **ergot alkaloids** or **oxytocin**

Adrenaline specifically reverses the antihypertensive effects of **adrenergic neurone blockers** with the risk of severe hypertension

Pharmacodynamic properties

Adrenaline is a naturally occurring catecholamine secreted by the adrenal medulla in response to exertion or stress. It is a sympathomimetic amine and a potent stimulant of both α- and β-adrenergic receptors

Rapid relief of hypersensitivity reactions to allergies or to idiopathic or exercise-induced anaphylaxis

Has a strong vasoconstrictor action through α-adrenergic stimulation, which counteracts the vasodilatation and increased vascular permeability leading to loss of intravascular fluid and subsequent hypotension, the major features in anaphylactic shock

Stimulates bronchial β-adrenergic receptors and has a powerful bronchodilator action

Alleviates pruritus, urticaria and angio-oedema associated with anaphylaxis

In resuscitation procedures it is used to increase the efficacy of basic life support

Increased systolic blood pressure, reduced diastolic pressure (increased at higher doses), tachycardia, hyperglycaemia and hypokalaemia

Fetal risk

Crosses the placenta. There is some evidence of a slightly increased incidence of congenital abnormalities

Injection of adrenaline may cause anoxia, fetal tachycardia, cardiac irregularities, extrasystoles and louder heart sounds

Usually inhibits spontaneous or oxytocin-induced contractions of the uterus and may delay the second stage of labour; if uterine contractions are reduced there may be uterine atony with haemorrhage

Parenteral adrenaline should not be used during the second stage of labour

Breastfeeding

Secreted in breast milk and should be avoided

BP
Amiodarone hydrochloride

Proprietary

Amiodarone Hydrochloride 50 mg/mL Concentrate for Solution for Injection/Infusion (Hameln Pharmaceuticals Ltd)

Amiodarone Injection Minijet 30 mg/mL (International Medication Systems (UK) Ltd)

Amiodarone (non-proprietary, see BNF for details)

Group
Cardiac arrhythmias

Uses/indications
Severe rhythm disorders not responding to other therapies or when other treatments cannot be used

Type of drug
POM

Presentation
Solution for injection

Dosage
IV amiodarone 300 mg (from a prefilled syringe or diluted in 20 mL glucose 5%) should be considered after adrenaline to treat ventricular fibrillation or pulseless ventricular tachycardia in cardiac arrest refractory to defibrillation

An additional dose of amiodarone 150 mg can be given by IV injection if necessary, followed by an IV infusion of amiodarone 900 mg over 24 h (BNF, 2011)

Route of admin
IV

Contraindications
Hypersensitivity to any of the excipients, e.g. iodine

Infants and children up to 3 years old

Severe respiratory failure, circulatory collapse, or severe arterial hypotension; hypotension, heart failure and cardiomyopathy are also contraindications if 50 mg/mL is given as a bolus injection

Evidence or history of thyroid dysfunction or cardiac conditions

NB: the above contraindications do not apply if cardiac arrest

Side effects
Infusion phlebitis, bradycardia, hypotension

Interactions
Due to the long and variable half-life of amiodarone (approximately 50 days), potential for drug interactions exists not only with concomitant medication but also with drugs administered after discontinuation of amiodarone

Warfarin, phenytoin, digoxin and any drug that prolongs the QT interval

Pharmacodynamic properties
A membrane-stabilizing antiarrhythmic drug that increases the duration of the action potential and refractory period in atrial and ventricular myocardium

Fetal risk
Crosses placental barrier

Most frequent complications include impaired growth, preterm birth and impaired function of the thyroid gland

Some evidence of hypothyroidism, bradycardia and prolonged QT intervals, increased thyroid gland or cardiac murmurs

Malformation does not appear to be increased, although cardiac defects need to be considered

Given the long half-life of amiodarone, women of childbearing age would need to plan for a pregnancy starting at least half a year after finishing therapy, in order to avoid exposure of the embryo/fetus during early pregnancy

Breastfeeding
If therapy is required during the lactation period or if taken during pregnancy, breastfeeding should be stopped

---

BP
Lidocaine

Proprietary
Lidocaine Hydrochloride Injection BP Minijet 1% w/v (International Medication Systems (UK) Ltd)
Lidocaine (non-proprietary, see BNF for details)

Group
Cardiac arrhythmias

Uses/indications
An alternative but only if amiodarone unavailable

After acute myocardial infarction it suppresses ventricular arrhythmias and reduces the potential for fibrillation and its recurrence. It decreases myocardial contractility and arterial blood pressure, and can be used where there is persistent ventricular fibrillation or ventricular tachycardia

Presentation
Minijet (Lidocaine Hydrochloride BP 10 mg/mL)

Dosage
100 mg as a bolus over a few minutes (reduced to 50 mg in lighter patients), followed by an infusion of 4 mg/min for 30 min, 2 mg/min for 2 h, then 1 mg/min; reduce concentration further if infusion continued beyond 24 h (ECG monitoring and specialist advice for infusion) (see BNF 2011 for guidance)

Route of admin
IV

Contraindications
Hypersensitivity to local anaesthetics of the amide type and in patients with porphyria

NB: continuous ECG monitoring is necessary during IV administration. Resuscitative equipment and drugs should be available immediately for the management of severe adverse cardiovascular, respiratory or central nervous system effects

CAUTION: epilepsy, liver disease, congestive heart failure, severe renal disease, marked hypoxia, severe respiratory depression, hypovolaemia or shock, and in patients with any form of heart block or sinus bradycardia. Hypokalaemia, hypoxia and disorders of acid–base balance should be corrected before treatment with lidocaine begins

Side effects
Allergic reactions (including anaphylaxis)
Light-headedness, drowsiness, dizziness, apprehension, nervousness, euphoria, tinnitus, blurred or double vision, nystagmus, vomiting, sensations of heat, cold or numbness, twitching, tremors, paraesthesia, convulsions, unconsciousness, respiratory depression and arrest, hypotension, cardiovascular collapse and bradycardia which may lead to cardiac arrest

Continued

Interactions
Propranolol and cimetidine may reduce the renal and hepatic clearance of lidocaine resulting in increased toxicity. The cardiac depressant effects of lidocaine are additive to those of other antiarrhythmic agents. Lidocaine prolongs the action of suxamethonium

Pharmacodynamic properties
Reduces automaticity by decreasing the rate of diastolic (phase 4) depolarization. Lidocaine is considered as a class 1b (membrane stabilizing) antiarrhythmic agent. The duration of the action potential is reduced due to the blockade of the sodium channel and the refractory period is shortened

Fetal risk
Safety has not been established, use if benefit outweighs risk

Breastfeeding
Caution as excreted in breast milk

BP
Sodium bicarbonate

Proprietary
Sodium Bicarbonate Injection BP Minijet 4.2% w/v (International Medication Systems (UK) Ltd)
Sodium Bicarbonate Injection BP Minijet 8.4% w/v (International Medication Systems (UK) Ltd)
Sodium Bicarbonate Intravenous Infusion (non-proprietary, see BNF for details)

Group
IV fluid

Uses/indications
Correction of metabolic acidosis associated with cardiac arrest after other resuscitative measures, e.g. cardiac compression, ventilation, adrenaline and antiarrhythmic agents, have been used

Type of drug
POM

Presentation
4.2% Minijet
8.4% Minijet
500 mL and 1000 mL packs for IV use
Sterile aqueous solution for injection

Dosage
Adults: the usual dose is 1 mmol/kg (2 mL/kg 4.2% solution or 1 mL/kg 8.4% solution) followed by 0.5 mmol/kg (1 mL/kg 4.2% solution or 0.5 mL/kg 8.4% solution) given at 10-min intervals
Or by continuous IV infusion of a weaker solution (usually 1.26%)
Emergency: 50 mmol if cardiac arrest is associated with hyperkalaemia (UK Resuscitation Council, 2010)
Premature infants and neonates: the 4.2% solution should be used or the 8.4% solution should be diluted 1:1 with 5% dextrose

Route of admin
Slow IV injection or continuous infusion

Contraindications
Administration of sodium bicarbonate is contraindicated in patients with renal failure, metabolic or respiratory alkalosis, hypertension, oedema, congestive heart failure, a history of urinary calculi and coexistent potassium depletion or hypocalcaemia, hypoventilation, chloride depletion or hypernatraemia

Side effects
Alkalosis and/or hypokalaemia may ensue as a result of prolonged use or over-correction of the bicarbonate deficit
Hyperirritability or tetany may occur, caused by rapid shifts of free ionized calcium or due to serum protein alterations arising from pH changes

Continued

Interactions

Caution should be used when administering sodium ions to patients receiving corticosteroids or corticotrophin

Urinary alkalization will increase the renal clearance of tetracyclines, especially doxycycline, but it will increase the half-life and duration of action of basic drugs such as quinidine, amphetamines, ephedrine and pseudoephedrine

Hypochloraemic alkalosis may occur if sodium bicarbonate is used in conjunction with potassium-depleting diuretics such as bumetamide, ethacrynic acid, furosemide and thiazides

Concurrent use in patients taking potassium supplements may reduce serum potassium concentration by promoting an intracellular ion shift

Pharmacodynamic properties

Sodium bicarbonate therapy increases plasma bicarbonate, buffers excess hydrogen ion concentration, raises blood pH and reverses clinical manifestations of metabolic acidosis

Fetal risk

Safe use in pregnancy has not been established risk/benefit needs to be assessed

Breastfeeding

Patients requiring IV sodium bicarbonate are unlikely to be fit enough to breastfeed, but recovery may alter outcome and breastfeeding could be initiated later

---

BP
Calcium gluconate

Proprietary
Calcium Gluconate BP (Hameln Pharmaceuticals Ltd)
Calcium Chloride (non-proprietary, see BNF for details)

Group
Electrolytes

Uses/indications

Cardiac resuscitation, acute hypocalcaemia, neonatal tetany
Acute colic of lead poisoning, as an adjunct in the treatment of acute fluoride poisoning and for the prevention of hypocalcaemia in exchange transfusions
NB: Calcium gluconate injection is used for the management of magnesium toxicity

Type of drug
POM

Presentation
Sterile injection

Dosage
Cardiac resuscitation: 7–15 mL (1.54–3.3 mmol)
NB: the absolute amount of calcium required for this indication is difficult to determine and may vary widely

Route of admin
IV infusion

Contraindications

Contraindicated in severe renal failure, hypercalcaemia (e.g. in hyperparathyroidism, hypervitaminosis D, neoplastic disease with decalcification of bone), severe hypercalciuria and in patients receiving cardiac glycosides

Side effects

If administered too rapidly, nausea, vomiting, hot flushes, sweating, hypotension and vasomotor collapse which may be fatal
Soft tissue calcification due to extravasation of calcium solutions has been reported
Adverse reactions have been reported in preterm and full-term newborns (aged <28 days) who had been treated with IV ceftriaxone and calcium

Interactions

Digoxin and other cardiac glycosides may be accentuated by calcium, and digitalis intoxication may be precipitated
Increased risk of hypercalcaemia with thiazides

Continued

Pharmacodynamic properties
Calcium is an essential body electrolyte
Essential for nerves, and muscle function and contraction, cardiac function and coagulation of the blood

Fetal risks
Should be used only if considered essential

Breastfeeding

Needs to be considered as excreted in breast milk

BP
Naloxone hydrochloride

Proprietary
Naloxone Hydrochloride Minijet® 400 mcg/mL
(International Medication Systems (UK) Ltd)
Naloxone Hydrochloride (non-proprietary, see BNF for details)

Group
Antagonist of central and respiratory depression

Uses/indications
Reversal of postoperative respiratory depression and reversal of neonatal respiratory and CNS depression resulting from opioid administration to mother during labour

Type of drug
POM

Presentation
Minijet, ampoules

Dosage
Term infant: 200 mcg single dose at birth or in divided doses of 10 mcg/Kg every 2-3 minutes (S.C. or IV)
Preterm infant: smaller dose agreed by paediatrician

Route of admin
IM, IV or S.C.

Contraindications
Hypersensitivity

Side effects

Abrupt reversal of narcotic depression may result in nausea, vomiting, sweating, tachycardia, hyperventilation, increased blood pressure, tremulousness and violent behaviour

In postoperative patients, larger than necessary doses of naloxone may result in significant reversal of analgesia and in excitement

Hypotension, hypertension, ventricular tachycardia and fibrillation, hyperventilation and pulmonary oedema have been associated with the postoperative use of naloxone

Seizures have occurred on rare occasions

NB: avoid use in neonates of opioid-dependent mothers as it can precipitate withdrawal symptoms and seizures

Interactions

Unless the stability of naloxone has been established, no drug or chemical agent should be added

Pharmacodynamic properties

An opioid antagonist that is devoid of the morphine-like properties of other antagonists. It acts within 2 min of IV administration but takes longer with IM or S.C. administration, although its effects via these routes last longer

Fetal risk

Crosses the placental barrier but no studies available on its use in pregnancy. Use only if needed

Breastfeeding

Use with caution

Drugs Used in the Treatment of Anaphylaxis

Anaphylaxis is a severe, life-threatening, generalized or systemic hypersensitivity reaction. It is characterized by the rapid onset of respiratory and/or circulatory problems and is usually associated with skin and mucosal changes; prompt treatment is required. In addition to the drugs listed below, the following is essential in the treatment of anaphylactic shock.

Oxygen

Oxygen is prescribed for hypoxaemic patients to increase alveolar oxygen tension and decrease the effort of breathing. Oxygen concentration depends on the condition being treated; the administration of an inappropriate concentration of oxygen can have serious or even fatal consequences.

Immediate initiation of high concentration oxygen therapy is required (usually more than 10 L/min) using a mask with an oxygen reservoir. Ensure high-flow oxygen to prevent collapse of the reservoir during inspiration. If the patient's trachea is intubated, ventilate the lungs with high-concentration oxygen using a self-inflating bag.

Intravenous fluids

Large volumes of fluid may leak from the patient's circulation during an anaphylactic reaction. Low blood pressure, vasoconstriction and signs of shock will be evident, so intravenous fluids need to be commenced immediately. There is no evidence to support the use of colloids over crystalloids; therefore, Hartmann's solution or 0.9% saline is suitable.

Bronchodilators

These include inhaled or intravenous **salbutamol**, inhaled **ipratropium**, intravenous **aminophylline** and/or intravenous **magnesium sulphate** (unlicensed).

BP   Adrenaline (epinephrine)
Proprietary   Adrenaline (Epinephrine) Injection BP 1 in 1000   (Hameln Pharmaceuticals Ltd)
Uses/indications   Anaphylaxis – see Adrenaline under cardiac arrest

BP
Hydrocortisone

Proprietary
Solu-Cortef® 100 mg (Pharmacia Ltd)
Hydrocortisone Sodium Succinate (non proprietary, see BNF for details)

Group
Corticosteroids

Uses/indications
In anaphylaxis (following initial resuscitation) is of secondary value in the initial management of anaphylaxis because the onset of action is delayed for several hours, but should be given to prevent further deterioration in severely affected patients
Suppression of the inflammatory response
Bronchial asthma (see manufacturers' information for other uses)

Type of drug
POM

Presentation
Ampoules – white, freeze-dried powder

Dosage
100–500 mg depending on severity of condition, administered by IV injection over a period of 1–10 min
This dose may be repeated at intervals of 2, 4 or 6 h as indicated by patient's response and clinical condition

Route of admin
IM, IV

Contraindications
Hypersensitivity to components and in systemic fungal infection. unless specific anti-infective therapy is employed
If live or live-attenuated vaccines are being used in patients receiving immunosuppressive doses of corticosteroids

Continued

Side effects

Unlikely as usually only used for short use

But side-effects attributable to corticosteroid therapy should be recognized (see manufacturers information)

Interactions

Drugs that induce hepatic enzymes enhance the metabolism of corticosteroids, so its therapeutic effects may be reduced, e.g. **rifampicin, rifabutin, carbamazepine, phenobarbital, phenytoin, primidone** and **aminoglutethimide**

Convulsions have been reported with concurrent use of **corticosteroids** and **ciclosporin**

Drugs that inhibit the CYP3A4 enzyme, such as **cimetidine, erythromycin, ketoconazole, itraconazole, diltiazem** and **mibefradil**, may decrease the rate of metabolism of corticosteroids and hence increase the serum concentration

Steroids may reduce the effects of anticholinesterases in myasthenia gravis

The desired effects of **hypoglycaemic agents, antihypertensives** and **diuretics** are antagonized by corticosteroids, and the hypokalaemic effects of acetazolamide, loop diuretics, thiazide diuretics and carbenoxolone are enhanced

Efficacy of **coumarin anticoagulants** may be enhanced by concurrent corticosteroid therapy and close monitoring of the INR or prothrombin time is required to avoid spontaneous bleeding

Renal clearance of **salicylates** is increased by corticosteroids, and steroid withdrawal may result in salicylate intoxication

Salicylates and **NSAIDs** should be used cautiously in conjunction with corticosteroids in hypothrombinaemia

Steroids have been reported to interact with neuromuscular blocking agents such as pancuronium, with partial reversal of the neuromuscular block

Pharmacodynamic properties
Anti-inflammatory action
When used in pharmacological doses, its actions reduce the clinical manifestations of disease in a wide range of disorders

Fetal risk
The ability of corticosteroids to cross the placenta varies between individual drugs; however, hydrocortisone readily crosses the placenta which in theory may result in hypoadrenalism in the neonate, although this usually resolves spontaneously following birth and is rarely clinically important

Breastfeeding
Excreted in breast milk, although no data are available for hydrocortisone

BP
Chlorpheniramine

Proprietary
Piriton® (GlaxoSmithKline Consumer Healthcare)
Chlorpheniramine Maleate (non-proprietary, see BNF for details)

Group
Antihistamine – sedative

Uses/indications
Emergency treatment of anaphylactic reactions
Adjunctive treatment following adrenaline for anaphylaxis
Symptomatic relief of allergy, e.g. hay fever, urticaria

Type of drug
POM

Presentation
Solution for injection

Dosage
Anaphylactic Reaction >12 years and adults: 10 mg IM or IV slowly (UK Resuscitation Council, 2010)
Antihistamine (symptom relief for allergy): see chapter 12

Route of admin

S.C., IM, IV

IV route is recommended in anaphylactic reactions in conjunction with emergency treatment, e.g. adrenaline (epinephrine), corticosteroids, oxygen and supportive therapy

Should be injected slowly over a period of 1 min, using the smallest adequate syringe

Contraindications

Hypersensitivity

In patients who have been treated with MAOIs within the last 14 days

Side effects

Slight drowsiness to deep sleep, difficulty concentrating, lassitude, blurred vision, nausea, vomiting and diarrhoea, urinary retention, headaches, dry mouth, dizziness, palpitation, painful dyspepsia, anorexia, hepatitis including jaundice, thickening of bronchial secretions, haemolytic anaemia and other blood dyscrasias

Allergic reactions including exfoliative dermatitis, photosensitivity, skin reactions and urticaria, twitching, muscular weakness and incoordination, tinnitus, depression, irritability and nightmares

Stinging or burning sensation at the site of injection.

Rapid IV injection may cause transitory hypotension or CNS stimulation

Interactions

Use with hypnotics/anxiolytics/alcohol may potentiate drowsiness

Inhibits phenytoin metabolism and can lead to phenytoin toxicity

Anticholinergic effects of chlorphenamine are intensified by MAOIs

Pharmacodynamic properties
Acts by competing with histamine for H_1-receptor sites on cells and tissues. Chlorphenamine also has anticholinergic activity

Fetal risk
Used only when the potential benefits outweigh the risks
Use during the third trimester may result in reactions in neonates

Breastfeeding
May inhibit lactation and may be secreted in breast milk
Use only when the potential benefits outweigh the unknown risks

Drugs Used in the Treatment of Severe Pre-Eclampsia and Eclampsia

BP
Magnesium sulphate heptahydrate (see BNF for details)

Proprietary
Magnesium Sulphate Injection BP Minijet 50% (International Medication Systems (UK) Ltd)
Magnesium Sulphate Injection, BP (non-proprietary, see BNF for details)

Group
Anticonvulsant – muscle relaxant

Uses/indications
Pre-eclampsia and eclampsia

Type of drug
POM

Presentation
Ampoules, Minijet

Continued

Dosage

Prevention of seizures in pre-eclampsia (unlicensed indication): initially IV injection over 5–15 min, 4 g followed by IV infusion, 1 g/h for 24 h; if seizure occurs, additional dose by IV injection, 2 g

Treatment of seizures and prevention of seizure recurrence in eclampsia: initially by IV injection over 5–15 min, 4 g, followed by IV infusion, 1 g/h for 24 h after seizure or delivery, whichever is later; if seizure recurs, increase the infusion rate to 1.5–2 g/h or give an additional dose by IV injection, 2 g

NB: for IV injection, concentration of magnesium sulphate heptahydrate should not exceed 20% (dilute 1 part of magnesium sulphate injection 50% with at least 1.5 parts of water for injections)

Route of admin
IV injection or infusion

Contraindications
Hepatic and renal impairment, hypersensitivity

Side effects
Hypermagnesaemia, nausea, vomiting, thirst, flushing of skin, hypotension, arrhythmias, coma, respiratory depression, drowsiness, confusion, loss of tendon reflexes, muscle weakness, and following oral administration colic and diarrhoea

OVERDOSE: loss of patellar reflexes, weakness, nausea, sensation of warmth, flushing, drowsiness, slurred speech, double vision

NB: according to BNF and manufacturer guidance, ECG monitoring and high-risk observations need to be taken to enable recognition of overdose

Interactions
Caution to patients receiving digitalis glycosides

Magnesium sulphate should **not** be administered together with high doses of **barbiturates**, **opioids** or **hypnotics** due to the risk of respiratory depression
the action of non-depolarizing muscle relaxants such as **Tubocurarine** is potentiated and prolonged by parenteral magnesium salts
Profound hypotension if used together with **nifedipine**

Pharmacodynamic properties
Magnesium is involved in neurochemical transmission and muscular excitability, and acts as a depressant on the CNS; peripherally causes vasodilatation. IV administration has an immediate effect that lasts for about 30 min

Fetal risk
Fetal heart rate should be monitored continuously; neurological depression of the neonate includes respiratory depression, muscle weakness and loss of reflexes

Breastfeeding
Secreted but considered safe

Antagonist
Calcium gluconate

BP
Diazepam emulsion

Proprietary
Diazemuls® (Actavis UK Ltd)

Group
Benzodiazepine – sedative, hypnotic, muscle relaxant

Uses/indications
Sedation prior to procedures such as endoscopy, dentistry, cardiac catheterization and cardioversion
Premedication prior to general anaesthesia
Control of acute muscle spasm due to tetanus or poisoning

Continued

Control of convulsions, status epilepticus
Management of severe acute anxiety or agitation
including delirium tremens

Type of drug
POM

Presentation
Emulsion

Dosage
Diazemuls® may be administered by slow IV injection
(1 mL/min), or by continuous infusion
Diazemuls® should be drawn into the syringe immediately prior to administration
Sedation: 0.1–0.2 mg diazepam/kg body weight by IV
injection. Normal adult dose is 10–20 mg, but dosage
should be titrated to patient's response
Premedication: 0.1–0.2 mg diazepam/kg body weight
by IV injection. Dosage should be titrated to patient's
response. In this indication, prior treatment with
diazepam leads to a reduction in fasciculations and
postoperative myalgia associated with the use of
suxamethonium
Status epilepticus: initial dose 0.15–0.25 mg/kg body
weight by IV injection repeated in 30–60 min if
required, and followed if necessary by infusion of up to
3 mg/kg body weight over 24 h
*Anxiety and tension, acute muscle spasm, acute states of
excitation, delirium tremens:* usual dose is 10 mg
repeated at intervals of 4 h, or as required
See manufacturer's guidance for further advice, e.g.
continuous infusion

Route of admin
IM, IV

Contraindications
Hypersensitivity to diazepam, benzodiazepines or any of the excipients, phobic or obsessional states, acute pulmonary insufficiency, myasthenia gravis, sleep apnoea, severe hepatic insufficiency, acute porphyria, use of monotherapy in patients with depression or those with anxiety and depression as suicide may be precipitated, hypersensitivity to egg or soybean **pregnancy and breastfeeding**

Side effects
Drowsiness, lightheadedness, confusion, **dependence**; after IV injection there may be a fall in blood pressure and severe respiratory depression; **overdose** – see manufacturer's guidance for detail

Interactions
Alcohol – enhances sedative effect
Anaesthesia – enhances sedative effect
Antiepileptics – reported both to increase and to decrease plasma phenytoin concentration
Antihistamines – enhanced sedative effect
Antihypertensives – enhanced hypotensive effect

Pharmacodynamic properties
Diazepam is a potent anxiolytic, anticonvulsant and central muscle relaxant, mediating its effects mainly via the limbic system as well as the postsynaptic spinal reflexes

Fetal risk
Teratogen in the first and second trimesters; prolonged use in the third trimester may cause neonatal respiratory depression, drowsiness, hypotonia and withdrawal Infants borne to mothers who took benzodiazepines chronically during the latter stages of pregnancy may have developed physical dependence and may be at risk of developing withdrawal symptoms in the postnatal period

Breastfeeding
Moderately safe in the short term but avoid repeated doses and observe the infant for lethargy and weight loss. With long-term use, see Fetal risk

References and Recommended Reading

Baxter, K., 2011. Stockley's Drug Interaction Companion. Pharmaceutical Press, London.

Briggs, G., Freeman, R., Yaffe, S., 2008. Drugs in Pregnancy and Lactation: A Reference Guide to Fetal and Neonatal Risk, eighth ed.. Lippincott Williams and Wilkins, Philadelphia.

Bubimschi, C., Weiner, C., 2010. Medication. In: James, D.K., Steer, P.J., Weiner, C.P., Gonik, B. (Eds.), High Risk Pregnancy: Management Options, fourth ed. Elsevier Saunders, London, pp. 579–598.

Centre for Maternal and Child Enquiries 2011. Saving Mothers' Lives, Reviewing Maternal Deaths to Make Motherhood Safer: 2006–2008. The Eighth Report of the Confidential Enquiries into Maternal Deaths in the United Kingdom. Available: http://www.oaa-anaes.ac.uk/assets/_managed/editor/File/Reports/2006-2008%20CEMD.pdf [accessed 2 March 2012].

Hofmeyr, G.J., Neilson, J.P., Alfrirevic, Z., Crowther, C., Duley, L., Gulmezoglu, M., Gyte, G.M., Hodnett, E.D., 2008. Pregnancy and Childbirth – A Cochrane Pocketbook. Wiley Cochrane Series, London.

Joint Formulary Committee, 2011. British National Formulary (BNF) 62. Pharmaceutical Press, London.

Jordan, S., 2010. Pharmacology for Midwives: The Evidence Base for Safe Practice, second ed. Palgrave Macmillan, Basingstoke.

Koren, G., 2007. Medication Safety in Pregnancy and Breastfeeding: The Evidence Based A–Z Clinician's Pocket Guide. McGraw-Hill, New York.

Paediatric Formulary Committee, 2011. BNF for Children 2011–2012. Pharmaceutical Press, London.

Rubin, P.C., Ramsey, M., 2007. Prescribing in Pregnancy, fourth ed. BMJ Books/Blackwell Publishing, Oxford.

Schaefer, C., Peters, P.W.J., Miller, R.K. (Eds.), 2007. Drugs During Pregnancy and Lactation: Treatment Options and Risk Assessment, Academic Press/Elsevier, London.

SPC from the eMC, Adrenaline (Epinephrine) 1:10 000 Sterile Solution, Minijet® International Medication Systems (UK) Ltd, updated on the eMC 26/10/05.

SPC from the eMC, Adrenaline (Epinephrine) Injection BP 1 in 1000, Hameln Pharmaceuticals Ltd, updated on the eMC 02/08/10.

SPC from the eMC, Amiodarone Hydrochloride 50 mg/mL Concentrate for Solution for Injection/Infusion, Hameln Pharmaceuticals Ltd, updated on the eMC 20/02/12.

SPC from the eMC, Amiodarone Injection Minijet 30 mg/mL, International Medication Systems (UK) Ltd, updated on the eMC 31/03/08.

SPC from the eMC, Calcium Gluconate BP, Hameln Pharmaceuticals Ltd, updated on the eMC 09/08/10.

SPC from the eMC, Diazemuls®, Actavis UK Ltd, updated on the eMC 10/06/11.

SPC from the eMC, Lidocaine Hydrochloride Injection BP Minijet 1% w/v, International Medication Systems (UK) Ltd, updated on the eMC 17/11/04.

SPC from the eMC, Magnesium Sulphate Injection BP Minijet 50%, International Medication Systems (UK) Ltd, updated on the eMC 07/11/05.

SPC from the eMC, Naloxone Hydrochloride Minijet® 400 mcg/mL, International Medication Systems (UK) Ltd, updated on the eMC 07/04/10.

SPC from the eMC, Piriton® tablets, GlaxoSmithKline Consumer Healthcare, updated on the eMC 28/05/10.

SPC from the eMC, Sodium Bicarbonate Injection BP Minijet 4.2% w/v, International Medication Systems (UK) Ltd, updated on the eMC 03/10/03.

SPC from the eMC, Sodium Bicarbonate Injection BP Minijet 8.4% w/v, International Medication Systems (UK) Ltd, updated on the eMC 19/02/09.

SPC from the eMC, Solu-Cortef®, Pharmacia Ltd, updated on the eMC 17/04/08.

UK Resuscitation Council, Resuscitation Guidelines 2010. Available: http://www.resus.org.uk/pages/guide.htm [accessed 19 May 2012].

Volans, G., Wiseman, H., 2012. Drugs Handbook 2012–2013, thirty-third ed. Palgrave Macmillan, Basingstoke.

16

Hypoglycaemics

These are agents that reduce the excessive level of glucose in the blood that is a feature of diabetes. Insulin and oral hypoglycaemics play a key role in the regulation of carbohydrate, fat and protein metabolism. Insulin is a polypeptide hormone of complex structure. There are differences in the amino acid sequence of animal insulins, human insulins and the human insulin analogues. Sources of insulin are bovine, porcine or human.

Insulin is a fuel-regulating hormone that controls the amount of glucose in the blood. People with diabetes have a deficiency of insulin and therefore a raised blood glucose level. Four types of insulin are available: fast, short, intermediate and long acting.

Women with insulin-treated diabetes who are planning to become pregnant must be informed that evidence is lacking about the use of long-acting insulin analogues during pregnancy. Therefore, isophane insulin (also known as NPH insulin) remains the first choice for long-acting insulin during pregnancy (NICE, 2008, p13).

Women with diabetes may be advised to use metformin or glibenclamide as an adjunct or alternative to insulin in the preconception period and during pregnancy, when the likely benefits from improved glycaemic control outweigh potential harm. All other oral hypoglycaemic agents (exenatide and liraglutide) should be discontinued before pregnancy and insulin substituted, as they cross the placenta and may cause severe hypoglycaemia in the neonate.

Hypoglycaemic therapy for women with gestational diabetes may include regular insulin, rapid-acting insulin analogues (aspart and lispro) and/or hypoglycaemic agents (metformin and glibenclamide) should be individualized to each woman.

Women who have been diagnosed with gestational diabetes should discontinue hypoglycaemic treatment immediately after the birth. Women with pre-existing type 2 diabetes who are breastfeeding can resume or continue to take metformin and glibenclamide immediately after birth, but other oral hypoglycaemic agents should be avoided while breastfeeding.

A medical diabetic consultant as well as a consultant obstetrician should care for women who have either insulin-dependent or gestational diabetes. Mixtures of insulin preparations may be required and appropriate combinations have to be determined for the individual patient.

The student should be aware of:

- the physiology and pathology of glucose metabolism
- the treatment of diabetes
- the methods for diagnosing 'gestational diabetes' and methods of treating the condition
- the sequelae of pregnancy complicated by diabetes
- local protocols for the care and treatment of mothers with diabetes during antenatal, intrapartum and postpartum periods, and during operative procedures such as LSCS (lower-segment caesarean section)
- care of the neonate after a diabetic pregnancy.

Short-Acting Insulin (Soluble)

- Usually administered 15–30 min before meals
- Effective after 30–45 min
- Peak effect after 1.5–4 h
- Duration 5–8 h

Rapid Acting Insulin

- Before or as soon as possible after meals
- Onset 5–20 min (depending on whether type 1 or 2 diabetes)

173

- Peak effect after 0.5–0.17 h (depending on whether type 1 or 2 diabetes)
- Duration 3–5 h

Intermediate Insulin

- Set times of the day
- Onset 1–2 h
- Peak effect 6–12 h
- Duration 12–24 h

Long-Acting Insulin

- Once daily, at same time
- Onset 2 h (may vary considerably)
- Peak effect 5–24 h (no peak)
- Duration 12–24 h

NB: Human preparations have more rapid onset and shorter durations.

When injected intravenously, soluble insulin has a very short half-life of about only 5 min and its effect disappears within 30 min.

BP
Insulin rapid acting

Proprietary
NovoRapid® (insulin aspart) (Novo Nordisk Ltd), Humalog® (insulin lispro) (Eli Lilly and Company Ltd), Apidra® (insulin glulisine) (Sanofi-Aventis)

Group
Rapid-acting analogue

Uses/indications
Insulin-dependent diabetes mellitus, insulin-dependent gestational diabetes

Type of drug
POM

Presentation
Varied: vial, cartridge, prefilled pen

Dosage
Dosing is individual and determined in accordance with the needs of the patient

Route of admin
S.C.
Some may be administered by continuous subcutaneous insulin infusion (CSII), intravenously or intramuscularly (see manufacturers' guidance)

Contraindications
Hypersensitivity to the active substance or to any of the excipients

Side effects
Hypoglycaemia, local reactions, fat hypertrophy at injection sites, anaphylaxis
Rarely: peripheral neuropathy
Uncommon: refraction disorders, diabetic retinopathy, lipodystrophy, oedema

Interactions
A number of other medicines may interact with insulin, e.g. oral antidiabetic agents, angiotensin converting enzyme (ACE) inhibitors, fluoxetine, monoamine oxidase inhibitors (MAOIs), salicylates and sulphonamide antibiotics, corticosteroids, diuretics, sympathomimetic agents (e.g. adrenaline (epinephrine), salbutamol, terbutaline), thyroid hormones, oestrogens, progestins (e.g. in oral contraceptives), protease inhibitors and atypical antipsychotic medicinal products (e.g. olanzapine and clozapine) and beta-blockers

Continued

Alcohol – enhances the hypoglycaemic effect

Analgesics – salicylates increase insulin requirements

β-blockers – enhance hypoglycaemic effect and mask warning signs, i.e. tremor

Corticosteroids – antagonize the hypoglycaemic effect

Contraceptives – antagonize the hypoglycaemic effect

Nifedipine – may cause impaired glucose tolerance

Smoking – may also antagonize the hypoglycaemic effect of insulin

Pharmacodynamic properties

The primary activity of insulins and insulin analogues is regulation of glucose metabolism. Insulins lower blood glucose levels by stimulating peripheral glucose uptake, especially by skeletal muscle and fat, and by inhibiting hepatic glucose production. Insulin inhibits lipolysis in adipocytes, inhibits proteolysis and enhances protein synthesis

Fetal risk

There are no adequate data on the use of the above in pregnant women

Healthcare professionals should be aware that data from clinical trials and other sources do not suggest that the rapid-acting insulin analogues (aspart and lispro) adversely affect the pregnancy or the health of the fetus or newborn baby (NICE, 2008, p13)

Breastfeeding

It is not known whether the above insulins are excreted in human milk, but in general insulin does not pass into breast milk and is not absorbed after oral administration

Breastfeeding mothers may require adjustments in insulin dose and diet

BP
Insulin short acting

Proprietary
Actrapid® (Novo Nordisk Ltd), Humulin S® (Eli Lilly and Company Ltd), Hypurin Bovine Neutral® (Wockhardt UK Ltd), Insuman Rapid® (Sanofi-Aventis)

Group
Short-acting insulin/neutral insulin

Uses/indications
As insulin rapid acting

Type of drug
POM

Presentation
Varied, e.g. vial, cartridge, prefilled pen, inhaler

Dosage
As insulin rapid acting

Route of admin
S.C.

Contraindications
Hypersensitivity to the active substance or to any of the excipients
Hypersensitivity to Humulin or to the formulation excipients, unless used as part of a desensitization programme
Under no circumstances should any Humulin formulation, other than Humulin S (soluble), be given intravenously
Hypoglycaemia

Side effects
As insulin rapid acting

Interactions
As insulin rapid acting

Pharmacodynamic properties
As insulin rapid acting

Continued

Fetal risk
As insulin rapid acting

Breastfeeding
As insulin rapid acting

BP
Insulin intermediate acting

Proprietary
Insulatard® (long acting) (Novo Nordisk Ltd), Humulin I®
(intermediate) (Eli Lilly and Company Ltd), Hypurin®
Bovine Isophane (intermediate) (Wockhardt UK Ltd)

Group
Medium- and long-acting insulin

Uses/indications
As insulin rapid acting

Type of drug
POM

Presentation
As insulin rapid acting

Dosage
As insulin rapid acting

Route of admin
S.C.

Contraindications
Hypersensitivity to the active substance or to any of the
excipients
Hypoglycaemia
Cardiac failure has been reported when pioglitazone
(oral hypoglycaemic) was used in combination with
insulin, especially in patients with risk factors for
development of cardiac heart failure
Hypersensitivity to Humulin or to the formulation
excipients, unless used as part of a desensitization
programme

Under no circumstances should any Humulin formulation, other than Humulin S (soluble), be given intravenously

Side effects
As insulin rapid acting

Interactions
As insulin rapid acting

Pharmacodynamic properties
As insulin rapid acting

Fetal risk
There are no adequate data on the use of the above in pregnant women

Breastfeeding
As insulin rapid acting

BP
Insulin (mixed insulin)

Proprietary
Humulin M3® (Eli Lilly and Company Ltd) – 30% Soluble insulin to 70% isophane insulin
Insuman Comb 25® (Sanofi-Aventis) – 25% dissolved insulin and 75% crystalline insulin

Group
Mixed insulin

Uses/indications
As insulin rapid acting

Type of drug
POM

Presentation
Vial, cartridge, prefilled pen

Dosage
As insulin rapid acting

Continued

Route of admin
Humulin M3® S.C. or IM (not IV)
Insuman Comb 25® S.C.

Contraindications
Hypersensitivity to Humulin or to the formulation excipients, unless used as part of a desensitization programme
Under no circumstances should any Humulin formulation, other than Humulin S (soluble), be given intravenously

Side effects
As insulin rapid acting

Interactions
As insulin rapid acting

Pharmacodynamic properties
As insulin rapid acting

Fetal risk
There are no adequate data on the use of the above in pregnant women

Breastfeeding
As insulin rapid acting

BP
Insulin long acting

Proprietary
Lantus® insulin glargine (Sanofi-Aventis), Levemir® insulin detemir (Novo Nordisk Ltd)

Group
Long-acting insulin analogue

Uses/indications
As insulin rapid acting

Type of drug
POM

Presentation
Various: vial, cartridge, prefilled pen (see manufacturers' guidance)

Dosage
As insulin rapid acting

Route of admin
S.C. (see manufacturers' guidance)

Contraindications
As insulin rapid acting

Side effects
As insulin rapid acting

Interactions
As insulin rapid acting

Pharmacodynamic properties
As insulin rapid acting

Fetal risk
There are no adequate data on the use of the above in pregnant women

Breastfeeding
As insulin rapid acting

BP
Metformin

Proprietary
Metformin hydrochloride (Aurobindo Pharma Ltd)
NOTE: unlicensed use in pregnancy

Group
Oral antidiabetic agent

Uses/indications
Type 2 diabetes

Type of drug
POM

Presentation
500 mg film-coated tablets

Continued

Dosage
Dosing is individual and determined in accordance with the needs of the patient

Route of admin
Oral

Contraindications
Hypersensitivity, diabetic ketoacidosis, diabetic pre-coma, renal failure or renal dysfunction, severe infection, shock, acute or chronic disease that may cause tissue hypoxia, such as: cardiac failure or recent myocardial infarction, alcoholism/alcohol intoxication, lactation

Side effects
Taste disturbance, nausea, vomiting, diarrhoea, abdominal pain and loss of appetite, erythema, pruritus, urticaria, lactic acidosis, decrease of vitamin B_{12} absorption

Interactions
Alcohol, iodinated contrast agents
care with glucocorticoids (systemic and local routes), β_2 agonists, and diuretics and ACE inhibitors

Pharmacodynamic properties
Metformin hydrochloride is a biguanide with antihyperglycaemic effects, lowering both basal and postprandial plasma glucose levels. It does not stimulate insulin secretion and therefore does not produce hypoglycaemia

Fetal risk
Manufacturers advise against use in pregnancy; however, NICE (2008) and BNF (2011) indicate strong evidence for its effectiveness and safety in pregnancy

Breastfeeding
Manufacturers advise against use in lactation; however, NICE (2008) and BNF (2011) indicate strong evidence for its effectiveness and safety in pregnancy

References and Recommended Reading

Baxter, K., 2011. Stockley's Drug Interaction Companion. Pharmaceutical Press, London.

Briggs, G., Freeman, R., Yaffe, S., 2008. Drugs in Pregnancy and Lactation: A Reference Guide to Fetal and Neonatal Risk, eighth ed. Lippincott Williams and Wilkins, Philadelphia.

Bubimschi, C., Weiner, C., 2010. Medication. In: James, D.K., Steer, P.J., Weiner, C.P., Gonik, B. (Eds.), High Risk Pregnancy: Management Options, fourth ed. Elsevier Saunders, London, pp. 579–598.

Fraser, R., Farrell, T., 2010. Diabetes. In: James, D.K., Steer, P.J., Weiner, C.P., Gonik, B. (Eds.), High Risk Pregnancy: Management Options, fourth ed. Elsevier Saunders, London, pp. 795–812.

Glibenclamide 2.5 mg tablets, Aurobindo Pharma Ltd, updated in BNF 62, 2011.

Hofmeyr, G.J., Neilson, J.P., Alfreirevic, Z., Crowther, C., Duley, L., Gulmezoglu, M., Gyte, G.M., Hodnett, E.D., 2008. Pregnancy and Childbirth – A Cochrane Pocketbook. Wiley Cochrane Series, London.

Joint Formulary Committee, 2011. British National Formulary (BNF) 62. Pharmaceutical Press, London.

Jordan, S., 2010. Diabetes mellitus and pregnancy. In: Jordan, S. (Ed.), Pharmacology for Midwives: The Evidence Base for Safe Practice, second ed. Palgrave Macmillan, Basingstoke, pp. 338–351.

Koren, G., 2007. Medication Safety in Pregnancy and Breastfeeding: The Evidence Based A–Z Clinician's Pocket Guide. McGraw-Hill, New York.

National Institute for Health and Clinical Excellence (NICE), 2008. Diabetes in Pregnancy. NICE, London.

Rubin, P.C., Ramsey, M., 2007. Prescribing in Pregnancy, fourth ed. BMJ Books/Blackwell Publishing, Oxford.

Schaefer, C., Peters, P.W.J., Miller, R.K. (Eds.), 2007. Drugs During Pregnancy and Lactation: Treatment Options and Risk Assessment, Academic Press/Elsevier, London.

SPC from the eMC, Actrapid®, Novo Nordisk Ltd, updated on the eMC 07/03/11.

SPC from the eMC, Apidra®, Sanofi-Aventis, updated on the eMC 04/05/11.

SPC from the eMC, Humalog®, Eli Lilly and Company Ltd, updated in BNF 62, 2011. on the eMC 13/05/11.

SPC from the eMC, Humulin I®, Eli Lilly and Company Ltd, updated on the eMC 01/08/11.

SPC from the eMC, Humulin M3®, Eli Lilly and Company Ltd, updated on the eMC 01/08/11.

SPC from the eMC, Humulin S®, Eli Lilly and Company Ltd, updated on the eMC 01/08/11.

SPC from the eMC, Hypurin® Bovine Isophane, Wockhardt UK Ltd, updated on the eMC 08/07/11.

SPC from the eMC, Hypurin® Bovine Neutral, Wockhardt UK Ltd, updated on the eMC 08/07/11.

SPC from the eMC, Insulatard®, Novo Nordisk Ltd, updated on the eMC 19/05/11.

SPC from the eMC, Insuman Comb 25®, Sanofi-Aventis, updated on the eMC 04/03/11.

SPC from the eMC, Insuman Rapid®, Sanofi-Aventis, updated on the eMC 04/03/11.

SPC from the eMC, Lantus®, Sanofi-Aventis, updated on the eMC 01/10/11.

SPC from the eMC, Levemir®, Novo Nordisk Ltd, updated on the eMC 13/01/12.

SPC from the eMC, NovoRapid®, Novo Nordisk Ltd, updated on the eMC 28/19/11.

SPC from the eMC, Metformin, Aurobindo Pharma Ltd, updated on the eMC 30/08/11.

Volans, G., Wiseman, H., 2012. Drugs Handbook 2012–2013, thirtythree ed. Palgrave Macmillan, Basingstoke.

Other Resources

Diabetes, U.K., Insulin wallchart. Available: http://www.diabetes.org.uk/Documents/Magazines/Insulinwallchart.pdf.

Acknowledgements

The authors wish to thank Janine Davis RGN, RM for her help in compiling this chapter.

17

Immunoglobulins

These are antibodies, present in the blood, that by specific and direct action defend the body against invading bacteria or organisms. Anti-D immunoglobulin is used prophylactically and in treatment of rhesus iso-immunization in women whose blood is rhesus negative. This immunoglobulin, given via injection, coats fetal cells that may have leaked into the maternal circulation following a sensitizing episode, thus preventing the woman becoming rhesus iso-immunized.

Some antibodies that are present in maternal blood require consultation with the Regional Blood Transfusion Centre as to their relevance to the mother and the fetus/neonate.

Other uses of immunoglobulins include those used as vaccines, i.e. hepatitis, varicella, rubella, tuberculosis, rabies and tetanus, some of which are discussed in Chapter 20.

The student should be aware of:

- blood grouping and rhesus evaluation
- the aetiology of Rhesus iso-immunization
- prevention of iso-immunization
- what action should be taken when there is a possibility that iso-immunization could occur, e.g. in antepartum haemorrhage
- counselling to prevent iso-immunization
- the sequelae to mother and fetus/neonate of rhesus iso-immunization
- the RCOG and NICE guidelines for administration of anti-D in pregnancy

- an awareness of other antibodies present in blood, e.g. Lewis, Kell, Duffy anti-E and anti-Fy, etc.
- the sequelae of infection by varicella zoster in pregnant mothers and neonates
- the administration of immunoglobulin to ameliorate the effects of such infection
- the RCOG guidelines for treatment of varicella zoster contacts.

When evaluating serum titres, the date of the last dose of anti-D should be included on the request document as the antibodies persist in circulation and may give a falsely high reading.

BP
Anti-D (Rh) immunoglobulin

Proprietary
D-GAM® Anti-D Rh Immunoglobulin (BPL) – available in 250 IU, 500 IU, 1500 IU and 2500 IU vials – doses according to haematologist instructions
Rhophylac® (CSL)

Group
Immunoglobulins – specific

Uses/indications
Prevention of RhD immunization in RhD-negative women:
- pregnancy/delivery of a RhD-positive baby
- abortion/threatened abortion, ectopic pregnancy or hydatidiform mole
- after antepartum haemorrhage (APH), amniocentesis, chorionic biopsy or obstetric manipulative procedure, e.g. external cephalic version, or abdominal trauma that may cause transplacental haemorrhage (TPH)
- treatment of RhD-negative patients after transfusion of RhD-positive blood or other products containing RhD-positive red blood cells (e.g. platelets)

Rhophylac® (CSL) – see BNF and SPC for detail

Type of drug
POM

Presentation
Solution for injection

Dosage
Postnatal dosage: the recommended dose is 500 IU as soon as possible within 72 h of delivery (additional doses of anti-D should be considered if a large fetomaternal haemorrhage (FMH) is suspected)
Antenatal prophylaxis: 500 IU given at both 28 and 34 weeks of gestation, or a single dose of 1500 IU at 28 weeks' gestation
Following a potentially sensitizing event during pregnancy: administered as soon as possible and no later than 72 h after the event

- up to 20 weeks' gestation: recommended dose is 250 IU per incident
- after 20 weeks' gestation: recommended dose is 500 IU per incident (a test for the size of the FMH should be performed when anti-D is given after 20 weeks and additional doses of anti-D should be administered as indicated)

Prevention of immunization in RhD-negative patients given blood components containing RhD-positive cells: recommended doses 125 IU per mL of transfused RhD-positive red cells
Students and midwives should consult the NICE Clinical Guidelines (CG37) Routine Postnatal Care of Women and their Babies (NICE, 2006)

Route of admin
D-GAM®, Human Anti-D Immunoglobulin deep IM, S.C. in haemorrhagic disease; also, if more than 5 mL volume doses should be divided and administered at different injection sites

Continued

Contraindications

Caution in those who have had an adverse reaction to blood transfusion or to administration of blood derivatives

Hypersensitivity

IM route is contraindicated in persons with severe thrombocytopenia or other disorders of haemostasis

Side effects

Soreness at injection site

Occasionally fever, malaise, headache and chills

Interactions

Live vaccines – if anti-D is given within 2–4 weeks of live vaccine then its action may be impaired

Pharmacodynamic properties

During a sensitizing episode when fetal cells enter the maternal circulation, if they are Rhesus D positive then the body treats them as foreign and makes antibodies against them. This is iso-immunization. When the mother comes into contact with RhD-positive cells again, either later in the same pregnancy or in subsequent pregnancies, her immune system produces immunoglobulins that cross the placenta and destroy fetal blood cells, causing haemolytic disease in the fetus. Anti-D coats fetal cells and disguises them from the maternal immune system so that either the mother remains non-immunized or her system is 'blind' to the fetal cells until they degrade naturally

Fetal risk

N/A

Breastfeeding

No data available

BP

Varicella zoster immunoglobulin

Proprietary

Varilrix® (GlaxoSmithKline UK)

Group
Immunoglobulins – specific

Uses/indications
Indicated for active immunization against varicella in healthy adults and adolescents (≥13 years) who are seronegative and at risk
Not indicated for routine use in children, it may be administered to seronegative healthy children 1–12 years of age who are close contacts (e.g. household) of persons considered to be at high risk of severe varicella infections

Type of drug
POM

Presentation
Powder and solvent to prepare solution for injection, vials of solution for injection

Dosage
Varilrix® (live vaccine): two doses (each of 0.5 mL reconstituted vaccine) should be given, with an interval between doses of at least 6 weeks but in no circumstances less than 4 weeks

Route of admin
S.C.

Contraindications
Hypersensitivity to neomycin, severe febrile state, those in an immunocompromised state, pregnancy and breastfeeding

Side effects
Acquiring chickenpox, headache, dizziness, nausea, muscle aches

Interactions
In individuals who have received immune globulins or a blood transfusion, vaccination should be delayed for at least 3 months

Continued

Care in children under 16 receiving aspirin and systemic salicylates because of the risk of Reye's syndrome

If a measles-containing vaccine is not given at the same time as Varilrix®, an interval of at least 1 month is recommended between administrations

If another live vaccine is given at the same time, separate injections at different body sites are essential

Pharmacodynamic properties
Infection of the subject with varicella zoster induces the humoral and cell-mediated immune response and thus immunity

Fetal risk
Manufacturers recommend that Varilrix® should not be given to pregnant women as this may cause the fetus to contract chickenpox, to be born with a (mild) form of chickenpox or scars from lesions

May cause respiratory tract problems

Breastfeeding
Women should not be vaccinated while breastfeeding

BP
Varicella zoster immunoglobulin

Proprietary
Human Varicella-Zoster Immunoglobulin (BPL)

Group
Immunoglobulins – specific

Uses/indications
Prophylaxis against varicella-zoster virus (VZV) infection in at-risk patients exposed to varicella (chickenpox) or herpes zoster:
- pregnant women with negative VZV immune status, especially up to early in the third trimester
- neonates whose mothers develop varicella infection within 7 days before and 7 days after delivery

- neonates whose mothers have no history of varicella and/or a negative immune status
- premature infants <28 weeks of gestation or newborns with low birthweight

Adults and children with no history of varicella and/or a negative immune status, receiving immunosuppressive therapy including steroids, cytostatic agents, radiotherapy, recent stem cell transplantation, or who have congenital or acquired immune deficiency disorders and are not receiving replacement therapy with immunoglobulin

Type of drug
POM

Presentation
Solution for injection

Dosage
Depending on age

Route of admin
IM

Contraindications
Hypersensitivity to any of the components
Hypersensitivity to human immunoglobulins

Side effects
Hypersensitivity, anaphylactic shock, headache, tachycardia, hypotension, nausea, vomiting, skin reaction, erythema, itching, pruritus, arthralgia, fever, malaise, chill and discomfort at site of injection

Interactions
Immunoglobulin administration may interfere with the development of an immune response to live attenuated virus vaccines, such as rubella, mumps and varicella, for a period of up to 3 months
May result in misleading positive results in serological tests

Continued

Pharmacodynamic properties
Human Varicella-Zoster Immunoglobulin contains mainly immunoglobulin G (IgG) with a specifically high content of antibodies against VZV

Fetal risk
Clinical experience with immunoglobulins suggests that no harmful effects on the course of pregnancy, or on the fetus and the neonate, are to be expected

Breastfeeding
No evidence to suggest unsafe

References and Recommended Reading

Baxter, K., 2011. Stockley's Drug Interaction Companion. Pharmaceutical Press, London.

Briggs, G., Freeman, R., Yaffe, S., 2008. Drugs in Pregnancy and Lactation: A Reference Guide to Fetal and Neonatal Risk, eighth ed. Lippincott Williams and Wilkins, Philadelphia.

Bubimschi, C., Weiner, C., 2010. Medication. In: James, D.K., Steer, P.J., Weiner, C.P., Gonik, B. (Eds.), High Risk Pregnancy: Management Options, fourth ed. Elsevier Saunders, London, pp. 579–598.

Hofmeyr, G.J., Neilson, J.P., Alfreirevic, Z., Crowther, C., Duley, L., Gulmezoglu, M., Gyte, G.M., Hodnett, E.D., 2008. Pregnancy and Childbirth – A Cochrane Pocketbook. Wiley Cochrane Series, London.

Joint Formulary Committee, 2011. British National Formulary (BNF) 62. Pharmaceutical Press, London.

Jordan, S., 2010. Drugs and the immune system. In: Jordan, S. (Ed.), Pharmacology for Midwives: The Evidence Base for Safe Practice, second ed. Palgrave Macmillan, Basingstoke.

Koren, G., 2007. Medication Safety in Pregnancy and Breastfeeding: The Evidence Based A–Z Clinician's Pocket Guide. McGraw-Hill, New York.

National Institute for Health and Clinical Excellence (NICE), 2006 CG37 Routine Postnatal Care of Women and their Babies. NICE, London.

National Institute for Health and Clinical Excellence (NICE), 2008. TA156 Pregnancy (Rhesus Negative Women) – Routine Anti-D (Review), Review proposal and decision 2011. Available: http://guidance.nice.org.uk/TA156 [accessed 26 March 2012].

Paediatric Formulary Committee, 2011. BNF for Children 2011–2012. Pharmaceutical Press, London.

Royal College of Obstetricians and Gynaecologists (RCOG), 2007 Chickenpox in Pregnancy. Greentop Guideline No. 13. RCOG, London.

Royal College of Obstetricians and Gynaecologists (RCOG), 2011. Clinical Greentop Guideline No. 22: Use of Anti-D Immunoglobulin for Rhesus Prophylaxis. RCOG, London.

Rubin, P.C., Ramsey, M., 2007. Prescribing in Pregnancy, fourth ed. BMJ Books/Blackwell Publishing, Oxford.

Schaefer, C., Peters, P.W.J., Miller, R.K. (Eds.), 2007. Drugs During Pregnancy and Lactation: Treatment Options and Risk Assessment, Academic Press/Elsevier, London.

SPC from the eMC, D-GAM®, Human Anti-D Immunoglobulin 500IU, BPL (Bio Products Laboratory), updated on the eMC 12/09/11.

SPC from the eMC, Human Varicella-Zoster Immunoglobulin, BPL (Bio Products Laboratory), updated on the eMC 27/07/09.

SPC from the eMC, Rhophylac®, CSL Behring UK Ltd, updated on the eMC 23/08/2011.

SPC from the eMC, Varilrix®, GlaxoSmithKline UK, updated on the eMC 16/01/12.

Volans, G., Wiseman, H., 2012. Drugs Handbook 2012–2013, thirtythird ed. Palgrave Macmillan, Basingstoke.

18

Intravenous Fluids

Solutions of electrolytes and water are given intravenously, to meet normal fluid and electrolyte requirements or to replenish substantial deficits or continuing losses, when the patient is unable to take adequate amounts by mouth, e.g. nauseous, vomiting, haemorrhaging, dehydrated or ketotic.

The causes and severity of the electrolyte imbalance must be assessed from the clinical history and biochemical investigations. Sodium, potassium, chloride, magnesium, phosphate and water depletion can occur singly and in combination with or without disturbances of the acid–base balance. Actions must be taken to ensure that circulatory overload does not occur as a result of intravenous fluid therapy, as overloading will result in pulmonary oedema and breathlessness, which may cause respiratory arrest. Hence a record of all fluids infused is essential.

Plasma volume expanders are used for the treatment of circulatory shock, e.g. massive obstetric haemorrhage or where there is a sudden acute blood or plasma loss leading to a fall in blood pressure and resulting in blood cells collapsing while trying to redress their balance. They restore vascular volume, stabilizing circulatory haemodynamics and maintaining tissue perfusion.

Drugs should **NOT** be added to infusions of sodium bicarbonate, amino acids, mannitol, blood products or specially prepared fat emulsions, such as those used in neonatal intensive care units for feeding neonates (total parenteral nutrition) via the intravenous route.

Instructions regarding storage and degradation of solutions should be noted, and any deviation either from instructions or within the solution should indicate that the infusion should not be commenced, or, if in progress, should be discontinued.

Additive labels should be used to indicate what has been added to the solution, time, strength and, if relevant, expiry time/date, as well as patient identity and the signature of the practitioners checking the infusion. The practitioner must also be aware of the suitability of the additive to the electrolyte solution and where to refer any enquiries.

NB: All fluids should accurately reflect daily requirements, and close monitoring is required to avoid fluid and electrolyte imbalance.

Intravenous fluids are commonly described as crystalloids and colloids.

Crystalloids

These are solutions with small molecules that flow easily from the bloodstream into the cells and tissues. They contain similar concentrations of osmotically active particles to extracellular fluid, so fluid does not shift between the extracellular and intracellular areas. Crystalloids can be described as:

- **Isotonic** – with a concentration of dissolved particles equal to that of intracellular fluid. Osmotic pressure is therefore the same inside and outside the cells, so they neither shrink nor swell with fluid movement.
- **Hypotonic** – less concentrated than extracellular fluid, so fluid moves from the bloodstream into the cells, causing cells to swell
- **Hypertonic** – more highly concentrated than extracellular fluid, so fluid is pulled into the bloodstream from the cells, causing cells to shrink.

Intravenous crystalloid fluids in common use

Sodium chloride 0.9% This isotonic solution provides the most important extracellular ions in near physiological concentrations and is indicated in *sodium depletion,* used in fluid replacement and electrolyte balance, as an IV infusion, as a carrier for injections in which the prescribed drug requires reconstitution, or as a 'flush' for IV cannulae.

Cautions: impaired renal function, cardiac failure, hypertension, peripheral and pulmonary oedema, toxaemia of pregnancy.

Side effects: administration of large doses may give rise to sodium accumulation, oedema and hyperchloraemic acidosis.

NOTE: The term 'normal saline' should not be used to describe sodium chloride intravenous infusion 0.9%; the term 'physiological saline' is satisfactory, but it is preferable to state the actual composition of the fluid, i.e. sodium chloride intravenous infusion 0.9%.

Glucose solutions These are used mostly to replace water deficit and should not be given alone as they may lead to hyponatraemia and other electrolyte disturbances.

Sodium chloride and glucose These hypertonic solutions are indicated when there is combined *water and sodium depletion.* A 1:1 mixture of isotonic sodium chloride and 5% glucose allows some of the water (free of sodium) to enter body cells, which suffer most from dehydration, while the sodium salt with a volume of water determined by the normal plasma Na⁺ remains extracellular.

Glucose 5% This is used as an isotonic intravenous infusion (IVI) for fluid replacement, dehydration and when there is an insulin infusion for the prevention of diabetic ketoacidosis, i.e. during diabetic labours and to provide energy. **NB:** There are a number of different concentrations, i.e. 2.5% and 4% glucose in sodium chloride.

Cautions: becomes hypotonic when the glucose is metabolized; not to be used in resuscitation as can cause hyperglycaemia; care with cardiac and renal disease; and prolonged use does not provide enough daily calories.

Dextrose saline This hypertonic solution of sodium chloride 0.18% plus glucose 4% is contraindicated in hyperemesis due to an increased risk of Wernicke's encephalopathy. If it is necessary to balance electrolytes then give thiamine first and refer to BNF for dosage.

Side effects: hypertonic glucose injections may have a low pH and may cause venous irritation and thrombophlebitis.

Hartmann's solution (compound sodium lactate solution) This isotonic solution, used as an IVI to replace fluid and restore electrolyte balance, can be utilized instead of isotonic sodium chloride solution during or after surgery, or in the initial management of the injured or wounded; it may reduce the risk of hyperchloraemic acidosis. Often used in obstetrics as a carrier for syntocinon infusions or for 'preloading' before and during epidural analgesia.

Water for injection This is used to reconstitute drugs prescribed as IVI injection.

Intravenous potassium Potassium directly affects how well the body's cells, nerves and muscles function, hence maintaining its balance is essential.

Care must be taken when administering potassium as it is toxic to the heart and so must be given slowly except in extreme circumstances. Hypokalaemia may result if there is renal impairment. Careful patient monitoring is required. Intravenous pumps should be used to control the rate of administration.

Potassium chloride + glucose This is used in severe electrolyte depletion – exact regimen specified by the prescriber.

Potassium chloride + sodium chloride As above. Where possible, premixed infusion solutions should be used or, alternatively, potassium chloride concentrate, as ampoules containing 1.5 g (K^+ 20 mmol) in 10 mL, is **mixed thoroughly** with 500 mL sodium chloride 0.9% intravenous infusion. **NB:** Ensure additive label applied.

Potassium chloride + glucose + sodium chloride As above.

Colloids

These are also known as plasma expanders/expanders of the intravascular space. They pull fluid into the bloodstream and are used if the circulatory blood volume does not improve. The main concern with colloids is that they may enter the interstitium, resulting in the osmotic gradient being increased and thereby pulling additional water into the interstitium. Increased risk of endothelial injury and capillary leak are linked to thromboembolism, anaphylaxis and disseminated intravascular coagulation (DIC), conditions that often necessitate colloid therapy.

There are four main colloids: albumin, dextran, starches and gelatin.

Albumin Albumin is derived from human plasma. It is used to maintain normal oncotic pressure and to act as a carrier of some metabolites. Natural colloid, prepared from whole blood, contains soluble proteins and electrolytes but no clotting factors, blood group antibodies, or plasma cholinesterases. Albumin can be given without regard to the recipient's blood type.

Albumin solution (human albumin solution) This is a solution containing protein derived from plasma, serum or normal placenta; at least 95% of the protein is albumin. The solution may be isotonic (containing 3.5–5% protein) or concentrated (containing 15–25% protein).

Indications: usually used after the acute phase of illness, to correct a plasma volume deficit.

Cautions: history of cardiac or circulatory disease.

Contraindications: cardiac failure, severe anaemia.

Side effects: hypersensitivity reactions (including anaphylaxis) with nausea, vomiting, increased salivation, fever, tachycardia, hypotension and chills reported.

Isotonic solutions: human albumin solution 4.5%, human albumin solution 5%, Albunorm® 5%, Octalbin® 5% and Zenalb® 4.5%.

Concentrated solutions (20%): human albumin solution 20%, Albunorm® 20%, Flexbumin® 20%, Octalbin® 20%, Zenalb® 20%.

Dextran This is derived from glucose: Dextran 70 (BNF non-proprietary), RescueFlow® (Dextran 70 intravenous infusion 6% in sodium chloride intravenous infusion) – avoid in pregnancy.

Gelatin Gelatin is derived from a bovine source: Gelofusine®, Geloplasma® (manufacturer of Geloplasma recommends avoid at the end of pregnancy), Isoplex® and Volplex®.

Starches Hydroxyethyl starch (HES) is derived from amylopectin (a soluble polysaccharide).

■ Hetastarch (non-proprietary)
■ Pentastarch (non-proprietary), HAES-steril®, Hemohes®
■ Tetrastarch – Tetraspan®, Venofundin®, Volulyte®.

NB: It is not within the remit of this book to discuss blood products but it **MUST** be remembered that blood products are drugs and therefore the normal processes in relation to drug administration must be followed alongside the additional requirements set down in Trust policies and procedures.

References and Recommended Reading

Centre for Maternal and Child Enquiries 2011 Saving Mothers' Lives: Reviewing Maternal Deaths to Make Motherhood safer: 2006–2008. The 8th Report of the Confidential Enquiries into Maternal Deaths in the United Kingdom. Available http://www.oaa-anaes.ac.uk/assets/_managed/editor/File/Reports/2006-2008%20CEMD.pdf [accessed 2 March 2012].

Hofmeyr, G.J., Neilson, J.P., Alfreirevic, Z., Crowther, C., Duley, I.., Gulmezoglu, M., Gyte, G.M., Hodnett, E.D., 2008. Pregnancy and Childbirth – A Cochrane Pocketbook. Wiley Cochrane Series, London.

Joint Formulary Committee, 2011. British National Formulary (BNF) 62. Pharmaceutical Press, London.

Jordan, S., 2010. Pharmacology for Midwives: The Evidence Base for Safe Practice, second ed. Palgrave Macmillan, Basingstoke.

Roberts, J., Bratton, S., 1998. Colloid volume expanders: problems, pitfalls and possibilities. Drugs 55, 621–630.

Royal College of Nursing (RCN), 2006. Right Blood, Right Patient, Right Time: RCN Guidance for Improving Transfusion Practice. RCN, London.

Royal College of Obstetricians and Gynaecologists (RCOG), 2007. Blood Transfusion in Obstetrics. Greentop Guideline No. 47 RCOG, London.

Rubin, P.C., Ramsey, M., 2007. Prescribing in Pregnancy, fourth ed. BMJ Books/Blackwell Publishing, Oxford.

Scott, W., 2010. Fluids and Electrolytes Made Incredibly Easy! Lippincott Williams and Wilkins, London.

Volans, G., Wiseman, H., 2012. Drugs Handbook 2012–2013, thirty third ed. Palgrave Macmillan, Basingstoke.

19

Miscellaneous

This chapter contains the drugs that are used in midwifery and that do not come under any previous title. Specific pre-existing conditions, e.g. asthma, or pregnancy-related conditions, e.g. obstetric cholestasis, require pharmaceutical treatments that should be familiar to most midwives in clinical practice.

The student should be aware of

- the non-pregnant physiology and adaptations during childbearing
- the abnormal pathology of pre-existing medical conditions
- the abnormal pathology of pregnancy-related disorders
- the medical management of these conditions during pregnancy, local protocols, and guidance for medication and monitoring of these conditions during childbearing.

Some medications listed here are complementary/alternative medicines. A recognized and registered practitioner in the complementary therapy should prescribe any such preparation, just as with conventional medicine one would seek the advice of a doctor or pharmacist prior to taking a medicine.

The student is urged to examine Standard 37 of the Code (NMC, 2008) and Standard 23 from the Standards for Medicines Management (NMC, 2007, updated 2010) on complementary and alternative therapies. Specific consideration of these sources is vital before considering the use of alternative or complementary therapies in any aspect of practice.

BP
Zidovudine (azidothymidine, sometimes known as AZT – abbreviation to be used with caution as it is also used for another drug)

Proprietary
Zidovudine (Aurobindo Pharma Ltd)
Retrovir® (ViiV Healthcare UK Ltd)

Group
Antiviral

Uses/indications
Management of HIV, possibly in the prevention of maternofetal HIV transmission

Type of drug
POM

Presentation
Capsules (white/blue band and blue-white/dark blue band), syrup 100 mg/10 mL
Powder for reconstitution, vials 200 mg in 20 mL solution (10 mg/mL)

Dosage
Prevention of maternofetal transmission (over 14 weeks' gestation): oral – 100 mg 5 times a day until labour
Labour and delivery: IV infusion at 2 mg/kg over 1 h, then 1 mg per kg per h until the cord is clamped. If LSCS planned, commence the regimen 4 h prior to delivery

Route of admin
Oral, IV infusion

Contraindications
Low haemoglobin or neutrophil counts, haematological toxicity: monitor blood levels
Vitamin B_{12} deficiency

Side effects
Multiple, including gastrointestinal disturbances, headache, rash, fever, anaemia

Interactions
Analgesics – methadone increases the plasma concentration of this drug

Antiepileptics – plasma phenytoin concentrations can increase or decrease; valproate – there is a potential for toxicity as plasma levels are increased

Pharmacodynamic properties
Antiviral agent that acts as a virostatic by disrupting viral DNA to inhibit growth and reduce viral numbers

Fetal risk
Use only if clearly indicated – possible maternal and fetal anaemia

Breastfeeding
Not recommended as HIV infection can be transmitted vertically

---

BP
Aciclovir (acyclovir)

Proprietary
Zovirax® (GlaxoSmithKlein UK)
Aciclovir (Pharmacia Ltd) (non-proprietary, see BNF for details)

Group
Antiviral

Uses/indications
Treatment of varicella-zoster in pregnancy, herpes zoster, shingles and cold sores

Type of drug
POM

Presentation
Powder for reconstitution, tablets, cream, cold sore cream, suspension

Dosage
Slow IV infusion over 1 h – 5 mg/kg t.d.s.
Oral: 800 mg × 5/day for 7 days

Topical: apply to lesion 4-hrly 5 times/day for 5–10 days – prompt recognition and commencement of treatment is recommended

Route of admin
IV infusion, oral, topical

Contraindications
Renal impairment

Side effects
Multiple, including rash, gastrointestinal disturbances, on IV infusion – local inflammation

Interactions
Ciclosporin and *tacrolimus* – increased risk of nephrotoxicity
Mycophenolate and *probenecid* – increased plasma concentration of aciclovir and metabolites of mycophenolate

Pharmacodynamic properties
A virostatic that interferes with the DNA reproduction function of the virus, reducing production and inhibiting its growth

Fetal risk
Use only when the benefits outweigh the risks, as the number of exposures to the drug is too limited to assess the long-term prognosis

Breastfeeding
Significant amount secreted into breast milk
Oral: 5-day course – considered safe
IV: insufficient information to allow classification as safe

BP
Thyroxine (levothyroxine sodium)

Proprietary
Eltorxin™ (Goldshield Group UK Ltd)
Thyroxine (non-proprietary, see BNF for details)

Group
Thyroid hormone

Uses/indications
Hypothyroidism

Type of drug
POM

Presentation
Tablets (25 mcg, 50 mcg, 100 mcg)

Dosage
As indicated by laboratory monitoring and the physician

Route of admin
Oral

Contraindications
Thyrotoxicosis, hypersensitivity

Side effects
These usually occur with overdose – tachycardia, palpitations, muscle cramps and other indications of an increased metabolic rate

Interactions
Antidepressants – tricyclics, amitriptyline – the antidepressant response is increased by the concurrent use of thyroxine
Anticoagulants – the effect of warfarin is enhanced
Antiepileptics – phenobarbital and phenytoin accelerate the metabolism of thyroxine; phenytoin levels are increased by thyroxine
Cimetidine – reduces the absorption of thyroxine from the gut
Cholestyramine – the absorption of thyroxine is reduced
Iron – ferrous sulphate – reduced absorption of thyroxine
Hypoglycaemics – monitor insulin requirements because of increased metabolic rate
Oral contraceptives – may increase plasma levels of thyroxine

Continued

Pharmacodynamic properties
A naturally occurring hormone that contains iodine and is produced by the thyroid gland – required for growth, development and the nervous system. It also increases the basal metabolic rate and has stimulatory effects on heart and skeletal muscle, liver and kidneys

Fetal risk
Monitor serum levels closely

Breastfeeding
Maternal dosage may interfere with neonatal screening for hypothyroidism

---

BP
Salbutamol

Proprietary
Ventolin™ Accuhaler™ (Allen & Hanburys Ltd)
Salbutamol (non-proprietary, see BNF for details)

Group
Selective β_2-adrenoceptor agonist – bronchodilator short acting

Uses/indications
Bronchodilator, immediate relief of asthma
Myometrial relaxant: see Chapter 18

Type of drug
POM

Presentation
Pressurized metered-dose inhaler

Dosage
100–200 mcg (1–2 puffs); for persistent symptoms up to 4 times daily; prophylaxis of allergen or exercise induced bronchospasm, 200 mcg (2 puffs)
duration of action 3–5 h
Premature labour: see Chapter 18 for regime if used as tocolytic

Route of admin
Inhalation

Contraindications
Placenta praevia, antepartum haemorrhage,
pre-eclampsia/eclampsia, threatened miscarriage,
hypersensitivity

Side effects
Fine tremor (particularly in the hands), nervous tension,
headache, muscle cramps
Palpitation, tachycardia, arrhythmias, peripheral vasodilata-
tion, myocardial ischaemia, hypotension, and collapse
Disturbed sleep and behavioural changes
Paradoxical bronchospasm (occasionally severe)
Urticaria, angio-oedema
High doses associated with hypokalaemia

Interactions
β-blockers, e.g. propranolol

Pharmacodynamic properties
Acts on β_2-adrenoceptors of bronchial muscle, with little
or no action on β_1-adrenoceptors of cardiac muscle

Fetal risk
Benefit should outweigh the risks; animal studies
indicate toxicity at high doses

Breastfeeding
Likely to be secreted in breast milk, so benefits should
outweigh risks

BP
Beclometasone dipropionate

Proprietary
Easyhaler® Beclometasone 200mcg (Orion Pharma UK Ltd)
Beclometasone (non-proprietary, see BNF for details)

Group
Corticosteroid

Uses/indications
Management of chronic asthma

Type of drug
POM

Presentation
Inhalation powder administered from multidose powder inhaler

Dosage
Maintenance: 200 mcg b.d.
Severe: starting dose may need to increase to 600–800 mcg per day and reduced once stabilized
Total daily dose may be administered as 2, 3 or 4 divided doses

Route of admin
Oral inhalation

Contraindications
Hypersensitivity
NB: special care in clients with active or quiescent pulmonary tuberculosis

Side effects
Candidiasis of the mouth and throat (clients are advised to rinse their mouth after using the inhaler)
Hoarseness/throat irritation, cough

Interactions
None reported

Pharmacodynamic properties
A pro-drug with weak glucocorticoid receptor binding activity, it is hydrolyzed via esterase enzymes to the active metabolite beclometasone-17-monopropionate (b-17-mp), which has high topical anti-inflammatory activity
NB: clients should be instructed in the correct use of the inhaler, and their technique checked, to ensure that the drug reaches the target areas within the lungs. The inhaler must be used regularly (even when asymptomatic for optimal benefit)

Fetal risk
Corticosteroids given to pregnant animals can cause abnormalities of fetal development including cleft palate and intrauterine growth restriction, hence a possible risk to the fetus
Manufacturer recommends use only if benefits outweighs risk

Breastfeeding
Recommend only if benefits outweighs risk

BP
Loperamide hydrochloride

Proprietary
Imodium® (McNeil Products Ltd)
Loperamide hydrochloride (non-proprietary, see BNF for details)

Group
Antidiarrhoeal

Uses/indications
Acute/chronic diarrhoea

Type of drug
POM

Presentation
Capsules/caplets, syrup, melts or instants

Dosage
Adjusted according to response: usually 4 mg initially and 2 mg after each loose stool thereafter to max dose of 12 mg in 24 h

Route of admin
Oral

Contraindications
Abdominal distension, acute ulcerative colitis

Side effects
Abdominal cramps, urticaria

Continued

Interactions
No data available

Fetal risk
No reports found linking loperamide with either human or animal toxicity, although not advised during first trimester

Breastfeeding
Small amounts of loperamide may appear in breast milk; therefore not recommended in breastfeeding

---

BP
Dexamethasone

Proprietary
Dexamethasone 4 mg/mL injection (Merck Sharp and Dohme Ltd)
Dexamethasone tablets (500 mcg), solution (2 mg/5 mL) and injection (4 mg/mL) (non-proprietary, see BNF for details)

Group
Glucocorticoid (steroid)

Uses/indications
To promote fetal lung surfactant production under 36 weeks' gestation and where labour is imminent/probable; can also ameliorate the effects of cholestasis of pregnancy

Type of drug
POM

Presentation
Tablets, IM injection – ampoules

Dosage
RCOG Greentop guidelines 2010: IM 6 mg 12 h apart for 4 doses (do not repeat after max dose) to reduce risk of respiratory distress syndrome (RDS) from preterm birth between 24 and 34 weeks' gestation; effective from 24 h to 7 days after second dose

Route of admin
Oral, IM

Contraindications
Avoid in suspected chorioamnionitis, tuberculosis, porphyria

Side effects
Rarely anaphylaxis, hypersensitivity, flushing, puerperal rash, fluid retention with repeated doses

Interactions
Analgesics – increases the risk of gastrointestinal bleeding with aspirin and other NSAIDs
Antibiotics – erythromycin may alter the metabolism of corticosteroids
Anticoagulants – alters the effects of anticoagulants, so monitor blood levels closely
Antidiabetics – antagonizes the hypoglycaemic effects
Antiepileptics – phenobarbital, phenytoin and carbamazepine accelerate the metabolism of corticosteroids
Antihypertensives – antagonizes the antihypertensive effect

Pharmacodynamic properties
A glucocorticoid with complex actions, one of which is to promote the production of lung surfactant. It is used to good effect when premature birth is anticipated and ameliorates the effects of cholestasis during pregnancy by reducing serum oestrogen levels. As premature delivery is an outcome of this condition, it also contributes towards reducing neonatal mortality and morbidity

Fetal risk
Overdose can affect the adrenal development of the fetus and neonate, and may contribute to intrauterine growth retardation (IUGR); however, the benefits vastly outweigh the risks of administration

Continued

Breastfeeding

No data available – but considered moderately safe if the benefits outweigh the risks

NB: infants of mothers taking high doses of systemic corticosteroids for prolonged periods may have a degree of adrenal suppression

---

BP
Betamethasone

Proprietary
Betnesol® (UCB Pharma Ltd)

Group
Glucocorticoid (steroid)

Uses/indications
To promote fetal lung surfactant production under 36 weeks' gestation and where labour is imminent/probable

Type of drug
POM

Presentation
IM injection – ampoules

Dosage
RCOG Greentop guidelines 2010: IM 12 mg 24 h apart, i.e. 24 mg in total (once only) to reduce risk of RDS from preterm birth between 24 and 34 weeks' gestation; effective from 24 h to 7 days after second dose

Route of admin
IM

Contraindications
Avoid in suspected chorioamnionitis, tuberculosis, porphyria

Side effects
Rarely anaphylaxis, hypersensitivity, flushing, puerperal rash, fluid retention with repeated doses

Interactions

Analgesics – increases the risk of gastrointestinal bleed with aspirin and other NSAIDs

Antibiotics – erythromycin may alter the metabolism of corticosteroids

Anticoagulants – alters the effects of anticoagulants, so monitor blood levels closely

Antidiabetics – antagonizes the hypoglycaemic effects

Antiepileptics – phenobarbital, phenytoin and carbamazepine accelerate the metabolism of corticosteroids

Antihypertensives – antagonizes the antihypertensive effect

Pharmacodynamic properties

A glucocorticoid with complex actions, one of which is to promote the production of lung surfactant. It is used to good effect when premature birth is anticipated

Fetal risk

Fetal teratogenicity at organogenesis; overdosage can affect the adrenal development of the fetus and neonate, and may contribute to IUGR; however, the benefits vastly outweigh the risks of administration

Breastfeeding

Considered moderately safe as there are no controlled studies involving breastfeeding women and their infants

---

BP
Prednisolone

Proprietary
Prednisolone 1 mg tablet, 5 mg tablet (Wockhardt UK Ltd)

Prednisolone (non-proprietary, see BNF for details)

Group
Corticosteroid

Continued

Uses/indications
Suppress inflammatory and allergic response, e.g. asthma, immunosuppressive disorders, rheumatic disease

Type of drug
POM

Presentation
White tablet – centrally scored

Dosage
Lowest effective dose to be advised
Initial: 5 mg to 60 mg in divided doses with or after food, in the morning – often reduced within days, and then continued under medical supervision until symptoms reduce
Maintenance: 2.5 mg to 15 mg daily

Route of admin
Oral

Contraindications
Systemic infection, hypersensitivity to ingredients

Side effects
Adrenal suppression
Suppression of the inflammatory response and immune function, thus increases susceptibility to infections (enhanced severity)
Severe psychiatric adverse reactions
Avoid exposure to measles and chickenpox (or herpes zoster) – seek urgent medical advice, but continue medication regimen
Increased monitoring should be given for clients with diabetes, hypothyroid conditions, epilepsy or hypertension

Interactions
Anticoagulants: efficacy of coumarin anticoagulants may be enhanced or reduced
NSAIDs: gastrointestinal bleeding and ulceration, renal clearance of salicylates is increased, steroid withdrawal may result in salicylate intoxication

Antibiotics – lower plasma concentrations and enhance renal clearance

Vaccines – avoid as impaired immune response

Hypoglycaemic agents (including insulin), antihypertensives and diuretics – effects likely to be diminished owing to antagonistic effect

Sympathomimetics, e.g. ritodrine, salbutamol, salmeterol, terbutaline – increased risk of hypokalaemia for high-dose usage

Intrauterine device – potential for failure of contraception

Pharmacodynamic properties
Glucocorticoid with anti-inflammatory and immunosuppressive action

Fetal risk
Crosses the placenta – variable, but 88% of prednisolone inactivated during transport
Animal studies have shown cleft palate, intrauterine growth restriction, brain growth and development anomalies
Benefits should outweigh the risks

Breastfeeding
Excreted in small amounts in breast milk; monitor for signs of adrenal suppression in infant, although benefits of breastfeeding are likely to outweigh this risk

---

BP
Clomifene (clomiphene) citrate

Proprietary
Clomid® (Sanofi-Aventis)
Clomifene (non-proprietary, see BNF for details)

Group
Anti-oestrogen

Uses/indications
Anovulatory infertility

Continued

Type of drug
POM

Presentation
Tablets

Dosage
50 mg/day for 5 days after the onset of menstruation; if no ovulation occurs after the first cycle then 100 mg for 5 days – use for a **maximum** of three cycles and under the supervision of a specialist centre

Route of admin
Oral

Contraindications
Pregnancy, hepatic disease, abnormal uterine bleeding, ovarian cysts except polycystic ovaries
CAUTION – with uterine fibroids

Side effects
Menstrual symptoms, hot flushes, abdominal discomfort, withdraw if there are visual disturbances or ovarian hyperstimulation, hair loss, weight gain, rashes, dizziness, rarely convulsions

Interactions
None stated (SPC, 2010)

Pharmacodynamic properties
Non-steroidal agent that stimulates ovulation in a high percentage of appropriately selected clients

Fetal risk
Fetal loss, ectopic pregnancy, risk of multiple pregnancy, multiple effects on fetal development, including neural tube defects and trisomies, reported – although not supported by data from population-based studies and still being investigated – therefore pregnancy should be excluded before the next course is commenced

Breastfeeding
Not known to be excreted in breast milk, but thought to reduce lactation

Name
Witch hazel (*Hamamelis virginiana*)

Proprietary
Distilled Witch Hazel BPC (Boots Company PLC)

Uses/indications
Varicosities, perineal trauma, haemorrhoids, herpes lesions

Type of drug
Herbal remedy

Presentation
Liquid

Dosage
As directed by practitioner

Route of admin
Topical

Contraindications
Broken skin/dermal tissue

Side effects
Occasional hypersensitivity reactions

Fetal risk
Safety not established – not recommended

Breastfeeding
Safety not established – not recommended

Name
Calendula officinalis (Marigold)

Uses/indications
Perineal trauma, sore nipples, cystitis, thrush, herpes

Type of drug
Herbal remedy

Presentation
Ointment, infusion

Dosage
As directed by practitioner

Continued

Route of admin
Oral or topical

Breastfeeding
Possible risk of allergy that can cause anaphylaxis –
therefore considered moderately safe as there are no
studies showing increased adverse effects in breastfeeding infants

---

BP
Peppermint water

Uses/Indications
To ease colic/flatulence and abdominal cramps

Type of drug
Herbal remedy, also used in aromatherapy

Presentation
Herbal tea: to treat anaemia and mood swings
Herbal suspension/infusion: as indicated above
Essential oil: to treat nausea and vomiting

Dosage
As directed by practitioner

Route of admin
Oral, inhaled

Name
Arnica montana (Leopard's Bane or Wolf Bane)

Proprietary
Astrogel arnica gel (Bioforce UK Ltd)
Arnica 30c pillules (A Nelson & Co. Ltd)

Uses/indications
First-aid remedy in bruising and soreness, e.g.
episiotomy or other perineal trauma

Type of drug
Homeopathic remedy

Presentation
Tablet or suspension

Dosage
As directed by homeopathic practitioner

Route of admin
Oral

Fetal risk
Avoid unless recommended by specialist practitioner

Breastfeeding
No evidence to suggest unsafe

Name
Ursodeoxycholic acid (UDCA)

Proprietary
Ursofalk® 250 mg capsules (Dr Falk Pharma Ltd)
Urdox® 300 mg film-coated tablets (Wockhardt UK Ltd)
Ursodeoxycholic acid (non-proprietary, see BNF for details)

Group
Acts on biliary composition and flow

Uses/indications
Dissolution of bile acids/gallstones; reduces itching and ameliorates liver enzymes; used in treatment of intrahepatic cholestasis of pregnancy (IHCP)

Type of drug
POM

Presentation
Tablets, capsules, suspension

Dosage
Oral: 8–12 mg/kg daily (20–25 g/kg daily – is considered effective and safe)

Route of admin
Oral

Contraindications
Pregnancy

Continued

Side effects
Nausea, vomiting, diarrhoea, pruritus

Interactions
Antacids – these bind to bile acids in the gut and have a detrimental effect on mode of action of UDCA

Cholestyramine – binds to bile acids in the gut and has a detrimental effect on mode of action of UDCA

Oestrogens – oral contraceptives – increased bile cholesterol is released, theoretically increasing the effective dose of UDCA

Pharmacodynamic properties
Complex action, but when given orally UDCA dissolves bile acids in the biliary fluid and disperses them, reducing cholesterol and thus ameliorating the cholestasis

Fetal risk
Teratogenic in animal studies and manufacturers' advise avoidance during early pregnancy; however, the benefits may outweigh the risks in IHCP

Breastfeeding
Manufacturer advises avoidance, but in the absence of controlled study data it is considered moderately safe when treating IHCP

BP
Nicotine

Proprietary
Nicorette® (McNeil); Nicotinell® (Novartis Consumer Health); NiQuitin® (GlaxoSmithKlein UK) – various preparations (tablets, patches, lozenges, chewing gum, inhalator see BNF for details); Champix® (Pfizer Ltd) – varenicline; Zyban® (GlaxoSmithKlein UK) – bupropion hydrochloride

Group
Nicotine replacement therapy (NRT)

Uses/indications
Smoking cessation regimes where other interventions have not been successful and health benefits are predicted from behavioural change

Type of drug
POM, some preparations available on GSL – **not** Zyban® or Champix®

Presentation
Various – see BNF for detail

Dosage
Under guidance of specialist practitioner with counselling and support available
Zyban® 150 mg prolonged release film-coated tablets
Champix® 0.5 mg film-coated tablets; Champix® 1 mg film-coated tablets (black triangle)

Route of admin
Oral, inhalation, transdermal

Contraindications
Consider risk/benefit assessment before initiating treatment: cardiac conditions (acute myocardial infarction), stroke, renal disease, phaeochromocytoma, hyperthyroidism, other dependencies
Diabetes mellitus – can affect carbohydrate metabolism, thus blood sugar levels should be monitored more closely than usual
Atopic or eczematous dermatitis (due to localized patch sensitivity) – discontinue use and seek medical advice

Side effects
Smoking cessation (general): could suffer from asthenia, headache, dizziness, sleep disturbance, coughing or influenza-like illness. Also depression, irritability, nervousness, restlessness, mood lability, anxiety, drowsiness, impaired concentration and insomnia which may be related to withdrawal

Continued

Other: nausea, headaches, faintness, (nicotine) dizziness, coughing or influenza-like illness Anaphylactic reactions, sleep disorders including abnormal dreams and insomnia, tremor, palpitations, tachycardia, dyspnoea, pharyngitis, cough, nausea, vomiting, dyspepsia, abdominal pain upper, diarrhoea, dry mouth, constipation, sweating increased, allergic dermatitis, contact dermatitis, photosensitivity, arthralgia, myalgia, application site reactions, chest pain, pain in limb, pain, asthenia, fatigue, malaise Symptoms of **acute nicotine poisoning** include nausea, salivation, abdominal pain, diarrhoea, sweating, headache, dizziness, disturbed hearing and marked weakness. In extreme cases, these symptoms may be followed by hypotension, rapid or weak or irregular pulse, breathing difficulties, prostration, circulatory collapse and terminal convulsions
Management of overdose: stop therapy immediately and admit to hospital. Monitor vital signs and ECG, maintain airway, ventilation and oxygenation

Interactions
May possibly enhance the haemodynamic effects of adenosine

Pharmacodynamic properties
Nicotine, an alkaloid in tobacco products and a naturally occurring autonomic drug, is an agonist at nicotine receptors in the peripheral and central nervous system and has pronounced CNS and cardiovascular effects

Fetal risk
Safety not established; manufacturers recommend smoking cessation without pharmacotherapy wherever possible

Breastfeeding
Compounds secreted in breast milk; manufacturers recommend that the benefit should outweigh the risk from smoking to either mother or baby

References and Recommended Reading

Baxter, K., 2011. Stockley's Drug Interaction Companion. Pharmaceutical Press, London.

Betnesol® injection 4 mg/mL, UCB Pharma Ltd, updated in the BNF 62, 2011.

Briggs, G., Freeman, R., Yaffe, S., 2008. Drugs in Pregnancy and Lactation: A Reference Guide to Fetal and Neonatal Risk, eighth ed. Lippincott Williams and Wilkins, Philadelphia.

Bubimschi, C., Weiner, C., 2010. Medication. In: James, D.K., Steer, P.J., Weiner, C.P., Gonik, B. (Eds.), High Risk Pregnancy: Management Options, fourth ed. Elsevier Saunders, London, pp. 579–598.

European Medicines Agency (EMA), 2010. HMPC Assessment Report on *Hamamelis virginiana*. Ref: EMA/HMPC/114585/2008. EMA, London.

Hofmeyr, G.J., Neilson, J.P., Alfreirevic, Z., Crowther, C., Duley, L., Gulmezoglu, M., Gyte, G.M., Hodnett, E.D., 2008. Pregnancy and Childbirth – A Cochrane Pocketbook. Wiley Cochrane Series, London.

Joint Formulary Committee, 2011. British National Formulary (BNF) 62. Pharmaceutical Press, London.

Jordan, S., 2010. Thyroid disorders in pregnancy. In: Jordan, S. (Ed.), Pharmacology for Midwives: The Evidence Base for Safe Practice, second ed. Palgrave Macmillan, Basingstoke.

Koren, G., 2007. Medication Safety in Pregnancy and Breastfeeding: The Evidence Based A–Z Clinician's Pocket Guide. McGraw-Hill, New York.

Medicines and Healthcare products Regulatory Agency (MHRA). Available: http://www.mhra.gov.uk/ (for information on Arnica, Calendula and Peppermint Water).

Nursing and Midwifery Council (NMC), 2007. updated 2010 Standards for Medicines Management. NMC, London.

Nursing and Midwifery Council (NMC), 2008. The Code: Standards of Conduct, Performance and Ethics for Nurses and Midwives. NMC, London.

Paediatric Formulary Committee, 2011. BNF for Children 2011–2012. Pharmaceutical Press, London.

Royal College of Obstetricians and Gynaecologists (RCOG), 2010. Antenatal Corticosteroids to Reduce Neonatal Morbidity and Mortality. Greentop Guidelines No. 7. RCOG, London.

Rubin, P.C., Ramsey, M., 2007. Prescribing in Pregnancy, fourth ed. BMJ Books/Blackwell Publishing, Oxford.

Schaefer, C., Peters, P.W.J., Miller, R.K. (Eds.), 2007. Drugs During Pregnancy and Lactation: Treatment Options and Risk Assessment, Academic Press/Elsevier, London.

SPC from the eMC, Aciclovir, Pharmacia Ltd, updated on the eMC 03/08/01.

SPC from the eMC, Champix® 0.5 mg film-coated tablets, Champix® 1 mg film-coated tablets, Pfizer, updated on the eMC 6/2/12.

SPC from the eMC, Clomid®, Sanofi-Aventis, updated on the eMC 1/9/10.

SPC from the eMC, Dexamethasone® 4.0 mg/mL injection, Merck Sharp and Dohme Ltd, updated on the eMC 27/1/11.

SPC from the eMC, Easyhaler® Beclometasone 200 mcg, Orion Pharma (UK) Limited, updated on the eMC 23/02/12.

SPC from the eMC, Eltroxin™ tablets, Goldshield Group Ltd, updated on the eMC 9/12/10.

SPC from the eMC, Imodium® 2 mg capsules, McNeil Products Ltd, updated on the eMC 10/7/12.

SPC from the eMC, Prednisolone 1 mg tablet, 5 mg tablet, Wockhardt UK Ltd, updated on the eMC 31/3/08.

SPC from the eMC, Retrovir®, ViiV Healthcare UK Ltd, updated on the eMC 10/2/12.

SPC from the eMC, Urdox®, Wockhardt UK Ltd, updated on the eMC 13/4/11.

SPC from the eMC, Ursofalk®, Dr. Falk Pharma UK Ltd, updated on the eMC 7/2/12.

SPC from the eMC, Ventolin™ Accuhaler™, Allen and Hanburys Ltd, updated on the eMC 3/1/12.

SPC from the eMC, Zidovudine 100 mg (or 250 mg) capsules, Aurobindo Pharma Ltd, updated on the eMC 3/3/11.

SPC from the eMC, Zovirax®, 250 mg, 500 mg, GlaxoSmithKline UK, updated on the eMC 09/07/02.

SPC from the eMC, Zyban® 150 mg prolonged release film-coated tablets, GlaxoSmithKlein UK, updated on the eMC 22/3/11.

Volans, G., Wiseman, H., 2012. Drugs Handbook 2012–2013, thirtythird ed. Palgrave Macmillan, Basingstoke.

Further Reading

Andrews, J.I., 2010. Hepatitis virus infections. In: James, D.K., Steer, P.J., Weiner, C.P., Gonik, B. (Eds.), High Risk Pregnancy: Management Options, fourth ed. Elsevier Saunders, London, pp. 469–478.

Bewley, C., 2011. Medical disorders of pregnancy. In: Macdonald, S., Magill-Cuerden, J. (Eds.), Mayes' Midwifery, fourteenth ed. Baillière Tindall/Elsevier, Edinburgh, pp. 771–786.

Centre for Maternal and Child Enquiries, 2011. Saving Mothers' Lives, Reviewing Maternal Deaths to Make Motherhood Safer: 2006–2008. The Eighth Report of the Confidential Enquiries into Maternal Deaths in the United Kingdom. Available: http://www.oaa-anaes.ac.uk/assets/_managed/editor/File/Reports/2006-2008%20CEMD.pdf [accessed 2 March 2012].

Tiran, D., 2011. Complementary therapies in maternity care: responsibilities of the midwife. In: Macdonald, S., Magill-Cuerden, J. (Eds.), Mayes' Midwifery, fourteenth ed. Baillière Tindall/Elsevier, Edinburgh, pp. 207–216.

Watts, D.H., 2010. Human immunodeficiency virus. In: James, D.K., Steer, P.J., Weiner, C.P., Gonik, B. (Eds.), High Risk Pregnancy: Management Options, fourth ed. Elsevier Saunders, London, pp. 479–492.

Williamson, C., Girling, J., 2010. Hepatic and gastrointestinal disease. In: James, D.K., Steer, P.J., Weiner, C.P., Gonik, B. (Eds.), High Risk Pregnancy: Management Options, fourth ed. Elsevier Saunders, London, pp. 839–860.

20

Myometrial Relaxants

These drugs are sympathomimetics and relax uterine muscle, hopefully preventing premature labour. Their main use is to delay delivery until corticosteroid therapy is complete. Some are used as antagonists to oxytocin, which can cause hyperstimulation of the uterus during the induction or augmentation of labour. Their use is indicated between 24 and 34 weeks' gestation in uncomplicated cases. Other terminology used for this group of drugs is tocolytics (RCOG, 2011).

The student should be aware of:

■ what constitutes premature labour
■ local protocols for the management of premature labour
■ the sequelae of the action of these drugs on the mother and fetus.

| **BP** |
| Terbutaline |
| **Proprietary** |
| Bricanyl® injection (AstraZeneca UK Ltd) |
| Bricanyl® 5 mg tablets (AstraZeneca UK Ltd) |
| **Group** |
| Myometrial relaxant/bronchodilator |

Uses/indications

Selective β_2-adrenergic agonist for the relief of bronchospasm in bronchial asthma and other bronchopulmonary disorders

To arrest labour between 24 and 33 weeks of gestation in patients with no medical or obstetric contraindication to tocolytic therapy. The main effect of tocolytic therapy is a delay in delivery of up to 48 h

Type of drug

POM

Presentation

Ampoules, tablets

Dosage

Injection – 0.5 mg/mL

Tablets 5 mg

As per local protocols or the manufacturer's recommendations – use of syringe pump or controlled infusion device essential

Route of admin

IVI, S.C., IM, oral

Contraindications

Pre-existing ischaemic heart disease or with significant risk factors for ischaemic heart disease

Hypersensitivity

Any condition of the mother or fetus in which prolongation of the pregnancy is hazardous, e.g. severe toxaemia, antepartum haemorrhage, intrauterine infection, intrauterine infection, severe pre-eclampsia, abruptio placentae, threatened abortion during first and second trimester, or cord compression

Side effects

Tachycardia tremor, headache, palpitations paradoxical bronchospasm, an increased tendency to bleeding in connection with peripheral vasodilatation, caesarean section, nausea, myocardial ischaemia, hypokalaemia, hypersensitivity reactions including angio-oedema, bronchospasm, hypotension and collapse, arrhythmias, e.g. atrial fibrillation, supraventricular tachycardia and extrasystole, symptoms of pulmonary oedema, mouth and throat irritation, sleep disorder and behavioural disturbances, such as agitation and restlessness, hyperactivity, hyperglycaemia, muscle spasms, hyperlactacidaemia, urticaria, rash

Interactions

Beta-blocking agents (including eye drops), especially the non-selective ones such as propranolol, may partially or totally inhibit the effect of β stimulants. Therefore, Bricanyl® preparations and non-selective beta-blockers should not normally be administered concurrently

Use with caution in patients receiving other sympathomimetics

Hypokalaemia may result from β_2-agonist therapy and may be potentiated by concomitant treatment with xanthine derivatives, corticosteroids and diuretics

Pharmacodynamic properties

Selective β_2-adrenergic stimulant that inhibits uterine contractility

Fetal risk

Administer with caution during the first trimester of pregnancy

Breastfeeding

Secreted into breast milk, but any effects on the infant are unlikely at therapeutic doses

Transient hypoglycaemia has been reported in newborn

BP
Salbutamol

Proprietary
Ventolin™ for IV infusion (Allen & Hanburys Ltd)
Salbutamol 4 mg tablets (Actavis UK Ltd)
salbutamol (non-proprietary, see BNF for details)

Group
Myometrial relaxant/bronchodilator

Uses/indications
Relief of severe bronchospasm
Management of premature labour; to arrest uncomplicated labour between 24 and 33 weeks of gestation in
patients with no medical or obstetric contraindication
to tocolytic therapy

Type of drug
POM

Presentation
Ampoules (5 mg/5 mL), tablets (4 mg)

Dosage
Pre-term labour: Syringe pump or controlled infusion
device essential during infusion; the maternal pulse rate
should be monitored and rate adjusted to avoid
excessive heart rate above 140 beats/min
The volume of fluid infused must be minimized to avoid
the risk of pulmonary oedema, hence strict fluid balance
records must be kept
Regimen: start 10 mcg/min and increase at 10-min
intervals to max 10–45 mcg/min depending on
contraction strength, frequency or duration. Then,
slowly reduce to cessation of contractions
Maintained at the same level for 1 h and then reduced
by half at 6-hrly intervals
If labour progresses despite treatment, the infusion
should be stopped
Maintenance once contractions cease: Salbutamol™ tablets
4 mg given three or four times daily in divided doses

Route of admin
Oral, IM, IV/infusion (in 5% dextrose – can use NaCl
with diabetic patients)

Continued

Contraindications

Threatened abortion

Hypersensitivity to any of the components

Pre-existing ischaemic heart disease or those with

Significant risk factors for ischaemic heart disease

Side effects

Hypersensitivity reactions including angio-oedema, urticaria, bronchospasm, hypokalaemia, hypotension, collapse, tremor, headache, hyperactivity, tachycardia, palpitations, myocardial ischaemia, cardiac arrhythmias including atrial fibrillation, supraventricular tachycardia and extrasystole

Particular to the management of preterm labour with salbutamol solution for infusion

Nausea, vomiting, muscle cramps, peripheral vasodilatation, pulmonary oedema (patients with predisposing factors including multiple pregnancies, fluid overload, maternal infection and pre-eclampsia may have an increased risk of developing pulmonary oedema)

CAUTION: discontinue if signs of pulmonary oedema or myocardial ischaemia develop

Interactions

Ventolin™ solution for IV infusion should not be administered in the same syringe or infusion as other medications

Salbutamol and non-selective β-blocking drugs, such as propranolol, should not generally be prescribed together

Pharmacodynamic properties

A selective β-antagonist that acts upon receptors in the uterus and bronchi, causing them to relax and lessening contractility

Fetal risk

Little evidence; use with care

Breastfeeding

Probably secreted in breast milk; use with care

BP
Ritodrine hydrochloride

Proprietary
Yutopar® (Durbin)

Group
Myometrial relaxant

Uses/indications
Inhibition of uncomplicated premature labour between 24 and 33 weeks' gestation, or to delay delivery by up to 48 h to administer glucocorticosteroids and implement other measures for neonatal well-being. Less effective if cervix more than 4 cm dilated or rupture of membranes is confirmed

Type of drug
POM

Presentation
Ampoules 10 mg/mL, tablets 10 mg (yellow) used to maintain uterine quiescence only

Dosage
As per local protocols, syringe pump or controlled infusion device is essential, for example:
IV infusion: initially 50 mcg/min, increased gradually according to response by 50 mcg/min every 10 min until contractions stop or maternal heart rate reaches 140 beats per min; continue for 12–48 h after contractions cease (usual rate 150–350 mcg/min); max rate 350 mcg/min
IM: 10 mg every 3–8 h continued for 12–48 h after contractions have ceased; then by mouth (but see notes above), 10 mg 30 min before termination of IV infusion, repeated every 2 h for 24 h, followed by 10–20 mg every 4–6 h, max oral dose 120 mg daily

Route of admin
Oral, IM, IV (in 5% dextrose)

Continued

Contraindications
Cardiac disease and in patients with significant risk factors for myocardial ischaemia
Avoid in antepartum haemorrhage, intrauterine infection, intrauterine fetal death, placenta praevia, abruptio placentae, threatened miscarriage, cord compression, and eclampsia or severe pre-eclampsia

Side effects
Flushing, sweating, salivary gland enlargement; leucopenia and agranulocytosis on prolonged administration (several weeks), liver function abnormalities (including increased transaminases and hepatitis), palpitations, hypotension, increased tendency to uterine bleeding, pulmonary oedema, chest pain and tightness
If tachycardic over 140 b.p.m. – cease infusion
See Salbutamol

Interactions
Anaesthetics – potential hypotensive effect
β-blockers – inhibit the action of ritodrine
Corticosteroids – with a high dose of ritodrine and high dose of corticosteroids there is an increased risk of hypokalaemia
Loop diuretics and thiazides – risk of hypokalaemia
Sympathomimetics – concurrent use potentiates the effects of ritodrine
Theophylline – risk of hypokalaemia
CAUTION – when used IV in diabetic clients, glucose levels should be monitored and insulin regimens need adjusting accordingly

Pharmacodynamic properties
A β-mimetic that stimulates β_2 receptors, thereby reducing uterine contractility. It also acts to cause cardiac effects and peripheral vasodilatation at therapeutic doses

Fetal risk
Studies show increased risk of obstetric haemorrhage, intrauterine death and transient neonatal tachycardia; fail to show teratogenicity, but recommended to avoid during the first 16 weeks of gestation

Breastfeeding
Considered moderately safe, but limited data available

BP
Nifedipine

Proprietary
Adalat® (Bayer PLC)
Nifedipine (non-proprietary, see BNF for details)

Group
β_2 agonists, calcium channel blocker, hypotensive, vasodilator

Uses/indications
Myometrial relaxant, tocolysis and hypertension

Type of drug
POM

Presentation
10 mg soft orange capsules
10 mg tablets grey–pink (modified release)

Dosage
Tocolysis: 10 mg stat. sublingually, then 10 mg at 15-min intervals for 1 h or until contractions have ceased, then 60–120 mg/day via slow-release tablets (or as per local protocol) (maintenance dose 20–40 mg q.d.s.), max dosage 160 mg in 24 h
Effective in 30–60 min
Hypertension: see Chapter 9

Route of admin
Oral

Continued

Contraindications

Contraindicated in pregnancy before week 20, breastfeeding, hypersensitivity, pre-eclampsia, pre-existing hypotension with systolic below 90 mmHg, previous adverse reaction to calcium channel blockers, cardiac disease – congestive cardiac failure, hepatic dysfunction, aortic stenosis, cardiogenic shock, acute angina attack; should not be administered concomitantly with rifampicin

Side effects

Headache, palpitations, flushing, dizziness, oedema, hypotension, nausea and vomiting

CAUTION: stop treatment if ischaemic pain occurs within 30–60 min of administration

Treatment with short-acting nifedipine, i.e. during a crisis, can induce an exaggerated fall in blood pressure and reflex tachycardia, which may cause complications such as cerebrovascular accident/ischaemia or myocardial ischaemia

Rarely: abnormal liver function tests, congestive cardiac failure, transient hypoglycaemia, tachycardia, chest pain, ischaemia (retinal/cerebral), tinnitus, pruritus

An increase in perinatal asphyxia, caesarean delivery, prematurity and intrauterine growth restriction, although unclear whether this is due to underlying hypertension, its treatment, or to a specific drug effect

EXTREME CAUTION when using magnesium sulphate

Interactions

Do not take with grapefruit juice

Antihypertensives – cause severe hypotension and possible heart failure

Cimetidine – potentiates the hypotensive effect as metabolism of nifedipine is inhibited

Phenytoin – concomitant administration can reduce the effect of nifedipine – monitor plasma levels of anticonvulsants

Erythromycin – may potentiate nifedipine effects

Insulin – possible impaired glucose tolerance

Pharmacodynamic properties

A selective calcium channel blocker with mostly vascular effects. It is a specific and potent calcium antagonist which relaxes arterial smooth muscle, causing arteries to widen and reducing the resistance in coronary and peripheral circulation. This reduces blood pressure and decreases the heart's overall workload

Fetal risk

Toxicity in animals, hypertensive effect can reduce placental flow and cause decrease in fetal oxygenation, i.e. *there is the potential for fetal hypoxia in association with maternal hypotension*

Contraindicated in suspected uterine infection, labour in the presence of placenta praevia, severe intrauterine growth restriction, lethal anomalies or fetal death in utero

Breastfeeding

Should be discontinued if nifedipine treatment becomes necessary during the breastfeeding period

Other medication that may be used include:

Tractocile 7.5 mg/ml Solution for Injection (Atosiban) (Ferring Pharmaceuticals Ltd) - see RCOG Greentop Guideline No 1b, 2011 and BNF 62, 2011 for details.

References and Recommended Reading

Baxter, K., 2011. Stockley's Drug Interaction Companion. Pharmaceutical Press, London.

Briggs, G., Freeman, R., Yaffe, S., 2008. Drugs in Pregnancy and Lactation: A Reference Guide to Fetal and Neonatal Risk, eighth ed. Lippincott Williams and Wilkins, Philadelphia.

Bubimschi, C., Weiner, C., 2010. Medication. In: James, D.K., Steer, P.J., Weiner, C.P., Gonik, B. (Eds.), High Risk Pregnancy: Management Options, fourth ed. Elsevier Saunders, London, pp. 579–598.

Hofmeyr, G.J., Neilson, J.P., Alfreirevic, Z., Crowther, C., Duley, L., Gulmezoglu, M., Gyte, G.M., Hodnett, E.D. 2008. Pregnancy and Childbirth – A Cochrane Pocketbook. Wiley Cochrane Series, London.

Joint Formulary Committee, 2011. British National Formulary (BNF) 62. Pharmaceutical Press, London.

Jordan, S., 2010. Drugs decreasing uterine contractility: tocolytics. In: Jordan, S. (Ed.), Pharmacology for Midwives: The Evidence Base for Safe Practice, second ed. Palgrave Macmillan, Basingstoke, pp. 178–195.

Koren, G., 2007. Medication Safety in Pregnancy and Breastfeeding: The Evidence Based A–Z Clinician's Pocket Guide. McGraw-Hill, New York.

Royal College of Obstetricians and Gynaecologists (RCOG), 2011. Greentop Guideline No. 1b. Tocolysis for Women in Preterm Labour. RCOG, London.

Rubin, P.C., Ramsey, M., 2007. Prescribing in Pregnancy, fourth ed. BMJ Books/Blackwell Publishing, Oxford.

Schaefer, C., Peters, P.W.J., Miller, R.K., 2007. Drugs During Pregnancy and Lactation: Treatment Options and Risk Assessment. Academic Press/Elsevier, London.

SPC from the eMC, Adalat®, Bayer PLC, updated on the eMC 08/02/12.

SPC from the eMC, Bricanyl® injection, AstraZeneca UK Ltd, updated on the eMC 16/04/09.

SPC from the eMC, Bricanyl® tablets and syrup, AstraZeneca UK Ltd, updated on the 20/05/09 and 20/01/10 respectively.

SPC from the eMC, Salbutamol 4 mg tablets, Actavis UK Ltd, updated on the eMC 12/1/11.

SPC from the eMC, Ventolin™, Allen & Hanburys Ltd, updated on the eMC 03/01/12.

Volans, G., Wiseman, H., 2012. Drugs Handbook 2012–2013, thirty-third ed. Palgrave Macmillan, Basingstoke.

Wales, N., 2011. Pre-term labour. In: Macdonald, S., Magill-Cuerden, I. (Eds.), Mayes' Midwifery, fourteenth ed. Baillière Tindall/Elsevier, Edinburgh, pp. 831–839.

Yutopar®, Durbin, updated in the BNF 62, 2011.

21

Oxytocics

Oxytocics (uterotonics) are drugs used to stimulate uterine contractions, i.e. for induction of labour, acceleration of labour, in active management of the third stage, to halt postpartum haemorrhage (PPH) and to control bleeding due to incomplete abortion. In the UK, the oxytocics used are prostaglandins, oxytocin, ergometrine, mifepristone and carbetocin (Pabal®).

The student should be aware of:

- the physiology of labour
- reasons for prolonged, incoordinate labour/contractions
- the physical, psychological and chemical factors that could diminish contractions
- reasons to expedite delivery
- research pertaining to managed and physiological third stage of labour
- appropriate emergency action to be taken in the event of syntocinon overdose
- the local emergency protocol for postpartum haemorrhage
- the sequelae of oxytocin administration in mother and neonate
- local protocols for the induction and augmentation of labour, including contraindications to therapy, e.g. cord prolapse, cephalo-pelvic disproportion, malpresentation, placenta praevia, antepartum haemorrhage, and cautions in predisposition to uterine rupture, multiple pregnancy, grande multiparity, polyhydramnios, previous caesarean section
- the action of oxytocin, ergometrine and syntometrine.

BP
Ergometrine maleate

Proprietary
Ergometrine Injection BP 0.05% w/v (Hameln)
(Non-proprietary, see BNF for details)

Group
Oxytocic

Uses/indications
Ergometrine Injection is used in the active management of the third stage of labour and in the treatment of postpartum haemorrhage

Type of drug
POM

Presentation
Sterile injection

Dosage
500 mcg ergometrine in 1 mL

Route of admin
IM, IV

Contraindications
Not be used during the first or second stages of labour, or administered to patients with hypertension (including that of pre-eclamptic toxaemia), occlusive vascular disorders, severe cardiac liver or renal failure or sepsis. The product is also contraindicated in patients with a known hypersensitivity to ergometrine
Special care if given to patients with sepsis or Raynaud's disease

Side effects
Headache, dizziness, tinnitus, cardiac arrhythmias, palpitations, bradycardia, chest pain, coronary arteriospasm with very rare reports of myocardial infarction, hypertension, vasoconstriction, dyspnoea, pulmonary oedema, nausea, vomiting, abdominal pain and skin rashes

Interactions
The vasoconstrictor effects of ergometrine are enhanced by sympathomimetic agents. Halothane anaesthesia may diminish the effects of ergometrine on the parturient uterus

Pharmacodynamic properties
Causes sustained contractions of the uterus **within 7 min IM and almost immediately IV**
Sustained uterine contractions
Controls uterine haemorrhage

Fetal risk
Ergometrine use is restricted entirely to the third stage of labour, otherwise it is not recommended for use during pregnancy

Breastfeeding
Ergometrine use is restricted entirely to the third stage of labour, otherwise it is not recommended for use during lactation

---

BP
Ergometrine maleate with Oxytocin

Proprietary
Syntometrine® (Alliance Pharmaceuticals)

Group
Oxytocic

Uses/indications
To expedite placental delivery, to control haemorrhage

Type of drug
POM

Presentation
Ampoules

Dosage
One ampoule: ergometrine 500 mcg + 5 units oxytocin in 1 mL

Continued

Route of admin
IM

Contraindications
Pre-eclampsia, renal impairment, first and second stages of labour, hepatic, cardiac or pulmonary disease, previous adverse reaction

Side effects
Nausea, vomiting, headache, dizziness, tinnitus, chest pain, palpitations, vasoconstriction, myocardial infarction, pulmonary oedema, stroke

Interactions
Halothane anaesthesia may diminish the uterotonic effect of Syntometrine®. May enhance the effects of vasoconstrictors and prostaglandins

Pharmacodynamic properties
Combines the sustained oxytocic action of ergometrine with the rapid action of oxytocin to act on the smooth muscle of the uterus to expedite placental separation and to control bleeding from the site of placentation after delivery **Syntocinon acts in 2–3 min IM; ergometrine acts in 7 min IM or almost immediately IV**

Fetal risk
Causes sustained uterine contraction and restriction of placental blood flow, leading to lack of oxygen to the fetus. If given to the neonate by accident causes serious and possibly fatal multi-organ shutdown

Breastfeeding
Secreted in breast milk but considered moderately safe

BP
Oxytocin

Proprietary
Syntocinon® (Alliance Pharmaceuticals)

Group
Oxytocic

Uses/indications
Early stages of pregnancy as a adjunctive therapy for the management of incomplete, inevitable or missed abortion
Induction of labour for medical reasons; stimulation of labour in hypotonic uterine inertia; during caesarean section, following delivery of the child; prevention and treatment of postpartum uterine atony and haemorrhage

Type of drug
POM

Presentation
Ampoules (5 units, 10 units)

Dosage
Incomplete, inevitable or missed miscarriage: by slow intravenous injection, 5 units followed if necessary by intravenous infusion, 0.02–0.04 units/min or faster
For induction or acceleration of labour: according to Trust protocols
Prevention of postpartum uterine haemorrhage: usual dose is 5 IU slowly IV after delivery of the placenta. In women given syntocinon for induction or enhancement of labour, the infusion should be continued at an increased rate during the third stage of labour and for the next few hours thereafter
Treatment of postpartum uterine haemorrhage: 5 IU slowly IV, followed in severe cases by IV infusion of a solution containing 5–40 IU oxytocin in 500 mL of a non-hydrating diluent, run at the rate necessary to control uterine atony (BNF 62, 2011)

Route of admin
IM, IV infusion or slow IV injection

Continued

Contraindications

Not within 6 h of prostaglandin administration, intact membranes, hypertonic uterine contractions, mechanical obstruction to delivery, fetal distress, where vaginal delivery is inadvisable, oxytocin-resistant uterine inertia, placenta praevia, vasa praevia, placental abruption, cord presentation or prolapse, severe pre-eclampsia, cardiovascular disease, caution in grande multiparity or where there is predisposition to uterine rupture, polyhydramnios, in cases of intrauterine death (IUD) or meconium-stained liquor – avoid tumultuous labour as it may cause amniotic fluid embolism

Side effects

Uterine spasm, uterine hyperstimulation, antidiuretic causing water intoxication, hypernatraemia, nausea, vomiting, rashes, **anaphylaxis**, placental abruption, amniotic fluid embolism – where possible, exclude this diagnosis prior to start of therapy

Interactions

Anaesthetics – can potentiate the hypotensive effect and may cause arrhythmias; the oxytocic effect may be reduced
Prostaglandins – uterotonic effect potentiated

Pharmacodynamic properties

Synthetic form of the hormone oxytocin. It exerts a stimulatory effect on uterine smooth muscle, especially at the end of pregnancy, during labour and post delivery, and in the puerperium when receptors in the myometrium are increased. In low doses it causes rhythmic contractions, but in high doses it causes hypertonic, sustained contractions

Fetal risk

Based on the wide use of this drug and knowledge of its chemical structure and pharmacological properties, it is not expected to present a risk of fetal abnormalities when used as indicated

Fetal distress, asphyxia, IUD
Recent literature identified no correlation between
oxytocin in labour and neonatal hyperbilirubinaemia
(Sanchez-Ramos and Delke, 2010)

Breastfeeding
Considered safe in the newborn because it passes into
the alimentary tract where it undergoes rapid
inactivation

BP
Carbetocin

Proprietary
Pabal® (Ferring Pharmaceuticals Ltd)

Group
Oxytocic

Uses/indications
For the prevention of uterine atony following delivery of
the infant by caesarean section under epidural or spinal
anaesthesia

Type of drug
POM

Presentation
Clear colourless solution for injection

Dosage
1 mL Pabal® containing 100 mcg carbetocin –
administer only by IV injection, under adequate medical
supervision in a hospital
Must be administered slowly, over 1 min, only after
delivery of the infant by caesarean section. It should be
given as soon as possible after delivery, preferably
before removal of the placenta

Route of admin
IV

Continued

Contraindications

During pregnancy and labour before delivery of the infant, not for the induction of labour, hypersensitivity, hepatic or renal disease, pre-eclampsia, eclampsia, severe cardiovascular disorders and epilepsy

CAUTION: migraine and hyponatraemia

Side effects

Headache, tremor, hypotension, flushing, nausea, abdominal pain, pruritus, feeling of warmth, anaemia, dizziness, chest pain, dyspnoea, metallic taste, vomiting, back pain, chills and pain

Interactions

Specific interaction studies have not been undertaken; however, as carbetocin is closely related in structure to oxytocin, similar interactions cannot be excluded

Pharmacodynamic properties

Selectively binds to oxytocin receptors in the smooth muscle of the uterus, stimulating rhythmic contractions of the uterus and increasing the frequency of existing contractions which raises the tone of the uterus musculature

Postpartum carbetocin is capable of increasing the rate and force of spontaneous uterine contractions. The onset of uterine contraction following carbetocin is rapid, with a **firm contraction being obtained within 2min**

Fetal risk

Contraindicated in pregnancy

Breastfeeding

Small amounts secreted in breast milk

References and Recommended Reading

Baxter, K., 2011. Stockley's Drug Interaction Companion. Pharmaceutical Press, London.

Briggs, G., Freeman, R., Yaffe, S., 2008. Drugs in Pregnancy and Lactation: A Reference Guide to Fetal and Neonatal Risk, eighth ed. Lippincott Williams and Wilkins, Philadelphia.

Bubimschi, C., Weiner, C., 2010. Medication. In: James, D.K., Steer, P.J., Weiner, C.P., Gonik, B. (Eds.), High Risk Pregnancy: Management Options, fourth ed. Elsevier Saunders, London, pp. 579–598.

Centre for Maternal and Child Enquiries 2011 Saving Mothers' Lives: Reviewing Maternal Deaths to Make Motherhood Safer: 2006–2008. The 8th Report of the Confidential Enquiries into Maternal Deaths in the United Kingdom. Available http://www.oaa-anaes.ac.uk/assets/_managed/editor/File/Reports/2006-2008%20CEMD.pdf [accessed 2 March 2012].

Hofmeyr, G.J., Neilson, J.P., Alfreirevic, Z., Crowther, C., Duley, L., Gulmezoglu, M., Gyte, G.M., Hodnett, E.D., 2008. Pregnancy and Childbirth – A Cochrane Pocketbook. Wiley Cochrane Series, London.

Joint Formulary Committee, 2011. British National Formulary (BNF) 62. Pharmaceutical Press, London.

Jordan, S., 2010. Drugs increasing uterine contractility: Uterotonics (oxytocics). In: Jordan, S. (Ed.), Pharmacology for Midwives: The Evidence Base for Safe Practice, second ed. Palgrave Macmillan, Basingstoke, pp. 148–177.

Koren, G., 2007. Medication Safety in Pregnancy and Breastfeeding: The Evidence Based A–Z Clinician's Pocket Guide. McGraw-Hill, New York.

McGeown, P., 2011. Induction of labour and post-term pregnancy. In: Macdonald, S., Magill-Cuerden, J. (Eds.), Mayes' Midwifery, fourteenth ed. Baillière Tindall/Elsevier, Edinburgh, pp. 851–860.

Rubin, P.C., Ramsey, M., 2007. Prescribing in Pregnancy, fourth ed. BMJ Books/Blackwell Publishing, Oxford.

Sanchez-Ramos, L., Delke, I., 2010. Induction of labour and termination of previable pregnancy. In: James, D.K., Steer, P.J., Weiner, C.P., Gonik, B. (Eds.), High Risk Pregnancy: Management Options, fourth ed. Elsevier Saunders, London, pp. 1145–1168.

Schaefer, C., Peters, P.W.J., Miller, R.K. (Eds.), 2007. Drugs During Pregnancy and Lactation: Treatment Options and Risk Assessment, Academic Press/Elsevier, London.

SPC from the eMC, Ergometrine Injection BP 0.05% w/v, Hameln Pharmaceuticals Ltd, updated on the eMC 03/06/08.

SPC from the eMC, Pabal®, Ferring Pharmaceuticals Ltd, updated on the eMC 06/10/10.

SPC from the eMC, Syntocinon®, Alliance Pharmaceuticals, updated on the eMC 27/03/07.

SPC from the eMC, Syntometrine®, Alliance Pharmaceuticals, updated on the eMC 21/04/10.

Volans, G., Wiseman, H., 2012. Drugs Handbook 2012–2013, thirty third ed. Palgrave Macmillan, Basingstoke.

22

Prostaglandins (PGE$_2$)

Prostaglandins are hormones secreted by various body tissues, e.g. uterine and cardiac muscle, semen and the lungs. Prostaglandins are used to ripen the cervix and stimulate the uterus to contract, resulting in labour. Prostaglandins can be administered by a number of routes: vaginal, oral, intravenous, extra-amniotic and intracervical.

Students should be aware of:

- the indications for induction of labour
- local protocols for induction of labour – specifically the medication and dosage used
- the action of prostaglandins with respect to termination of pregnancy and the side effects
- use of the Bishop's Score in the induction of labour.

BP	Dinoprostone
Proprietary	Prostin E2® (Pharmacia Ltd)
Group	Prostaglandins
Uses/indications	Induction of labour – ripening of the cervix for labour when there are no fetal or maternal contraindications
Type of drug	POM

Presentation
Prostin E2 Vaginal Gel 1 mg
Prostin E2 Vaginal Gel 2 mg
Translucent, thixotropic gel (NICE 2008 does not recommend tablets, IV solution or extra-amniotic solution for induction of labour)
Where tablets are used:
Prostin E2 Vaginal Tablets 3 mg

Dosage
CAUTION: Prostin E2 gel is not a bioequivalent to Prostin E2 tablets
Dependent on parity, local protocols and Bishop's Score
Gel should be inserted high into the posterior fornix avoiding administration into the cervical canal
Primigravidas (unfavourable) (Bishop's Score of 4 or less): initial dose of 2 mg administered vaginally
In others: initial dose of 1 mg administered vaginally
In both groups: a second dose of 1 mg or 2 mg may be administered after 6 h as follows:

- 1 mg should be used where uterine activity is insufficient for satisfactory progress of labour
- 2 mg may be used where response to the initial dose has been minimal
- max dose 4 mg in unfavourable primigravida patients or 3 mg in other patients

The patient should remain recumbent for at least 30 min after administration
Tablet (one) should be inserted high into posterior fornix. A second tablet may be administered after 8 hours. Max 6 mg.

Route of admin
P.V. (not intracervical)

Contraindications
Hypersensitivity, if oxytocic drugs are contraindicated or where prolonged contractions of the uterus are considered inappropriate, e.g. caesarean section or majoruterine surgery, potential or obstructed labour, pelvic

inflammatory disease (unless adequate prior treatment), active cardiac, pulmonary, renal or hepatic disease
CAUTION: asthma or a history of asthma, epilepsy or a history of epilepsy, glaucoma or raised intraocular pressure, compromised cardiovascular, hepatic, or renal function, hypertension, in women with compromised (scarred) uterus and women aged 35 years or older

Side effects

Asthma, bronchospasm, cardiac arrest, hypertension, rash, diarrhoea, nausea, vomiting, fever, anaphylactoid and anaphylactic reactions including anaphylactic shock, back pain, uterine hypertonus, uterine rupture, abruptio placenta, pulmonary amniotic fluid embolism, rapid cervical dilatation, uterine hypercontractility with/without fetal bradycardia, fetal distress/altered fetal heart rate (FHR), neonatal distress, neonatal death, stillbirth, low Apgar score, warm feeling in vagina, irritation, pain, increased risk of postpartum disseminated intravascular coagulation

Interactions

Oxytocics – uterotonic effect enhanced, hence it is not recommended that these drugs are used together
If used in sequence, uterine activity **MUST** be monitored carefully

Pharmacodynamic properties

A prostaglandin of the E₂ series that induces myometrial contractions and promotes cervical ripening

Fetal risk

ABORTIFACIENT: exposure to fetal skin in utero causes fetal heart rate abnormalities and may predispose to neonatal jaundice

Breastfeeding

Considered moderately safe, but with extremely limited data on the consequences of administration in breastfeeding women

BP
Dinoprostone

Proprietary
Propess® (Ferring Pharmaceuticals Ltd)

Group
Prostaglandins

Uses/indications
Induction of labour – ripening of the cervix for labour when there are no fetal or maternal contraindications

Type of drug
POM

Presentation
A thin, flat semi-opaque polymeric vaginal delivery system which is rectangular in shape with radiused corners contained within a knitted polyester retrieval system

Dosage

10 mg vaginal delivery system
If there is insufficient cervical ripening in 24 h, the vaginal delivery system should be removed
Following the removal of the vaginal delivery system at least 30 min is recommended before oxytocin is commenced
Administration
PROPESS should be removed from the freezer immediately before insertion
The vaginal delivery system should be inserted high into the posterior vaginal fornix using only minimal water-soluble lubricants
Once inserted, the withdrawal tape may be cut, ensuring there is sufficient tape outside the vagina to allow removal. The end of the tape **MUST** not be tucked into the vagina as this would make it difficult to remove
The patient should remain recumbent for 20–30 min after insertion

Continued

Dinoprostone will be released continuously over a period of 24 h, hence it is important to monitor uterine contractions and fetal condition

Removal

Gentle traction on the retrieval tape

Removal stops further drug administration when cervical ripening is judged to be complete, e.g. onset of labour, once regular, painful contractions have been established. In multigravidas the vaginal delivery system should be removed irrespective of cervical state to avoid the risk of uterine hyperstimulation, spontaneous rupture of the membranes or amniotomy, uterine hyperstimulation or hypertonic uterine contractions, evidence of fetal distress, maternal systemic adverse dinoprostone effects such as nausea, vomiting, hypotension or tachycardia, at least 30 min prior to starting an intravenous infusion of oxytocin

Route of admin

P.V. (not intracervical)

Contraindications

When labour has started, with other oxytocic drugs, when strong prolonged uterine contractions would be inappropriate, e.g. previous major uterine surgery (caesarean section, myomectomy), cephalopelvic disproportion, fetal malpresentation, fetal distress, more than three full-term deliveries, previous surgery or rupture of the cervix, current pelvic inflammatory disease (unless adequate prior treatment has been instituted), hypersensitivity, placenta praevia or unexplained vaginal bleeding during the current pregnancy

CAUTION: asthma or a history of asthma, epilepsy or a history of epilepsy, glaucoma or raised intraocular pressure, compromised cardiovascular, hepatic or renal function, hypertension, in women with compromised (scarred) uterus and women aged 35 years or older

Side effects
Asthma, bronchospasm, cardiac arrest, hypertension, rash, diarrhoea, nausea, vomiting, fever, anaphylactoid and anaphylactic reactions including anaphylactic shock, back pain, uterine hypertonus, uterine rupture, abruptio placenta, pulmonary amniotic fluid embolism, rapid cervical dilatation, uterine hypercontractility with/ without fetal bradycardia, fetal distress/altered fetal heart rate (FHR), neonatal distress, neonatal death, stillbirths, low Apgar score, warm feeling in vagina, irritation, pain

Interactions
Prostaglandins potentiate the uterotonic effect of oxytocic drugs

Pharmacodynamic properties
Prostaglandin E_2 (PGE$_2$) is naturally occurring and found in low concentrations in most body tissues. Cervical ripening involves relaxation of the cervical smooth muscle fibres of the uterine cervix, which must change from a rigid structure to a soft, dilated to allow passage of the fetus through the birth canal
Involves activation of the enzyme collagenase, which is responsible for the breakdown of the collagen

Fetal risk
Only used in induction of labour

Breastfeeding
Not indicated for use during lactation

BP
Gemeprost

Proprietary
Gemeprost (Sanofi-Aventis) Cervagem (Sanofi-Aventis)

Group
Prostaglandin

Continued

Uses/indications
Medical induction of late therapeutic abortion; also used to ripen the cervix before surgical abortion, particularly in primigravidas

Type of drug
POM

Presentation
White to yellowish-white spindle-shaped vaginal pessary

Dosage
Gemeprost 1mg Pessary
Cervagem 1mg Pessary
Dependent on stage of pregnancy and indication:
Softening and dilatation of cervix – 1 pessary to be inserted into the posterior vaginal fornix 3h before surgery
Therapeutic termination of pregnancy – 1 pessary to be inserted into the posterior vaginal fornix 3-hrly to a maximum of 5 administrations; a second course of treatment may be instituted starting 24h after the initial commencement of treatment
If abortion is not well established after 10 pessaries, a further course of Gemeprost treatment is not recommended and alternative means should be employed to effect uterine emptying
Intrauterine fetal death – 1 pessary to be inserted into the posterior vaginal fornix 3-hrly up to a maximum of 5 administrations

Route of admin
P.V.

Contraindications
Hypersensitivity, impaired renal function, chronic obstructive airway disease, cardiovascular insufficiency, raised intraocular pressure, cervicitis, vaginitis; caution with previous uterine surgery or placenta previa, induction of labour or cervical softening at term

Side effects
Vaginal bleeding, mild uterine pain, nausea, vomiting, loose stools/diarrhoea, headache, muscle weakness, dizziness, flushing, chills, backache, dyspnoea, chest pain, palpitations, mild pyrexia, rarely uterine rupture, anaphylactic reactions have not occurred with gemeprost, but such reactions have very rarely been noted with other prostaglandins; severe hypotension and coronary spasms with resulting myocardial infarction has been reported rarely

NB: careful monitoring of blood pressure and pulse essential for 3 h after administration due to risk of profound hypotension

Interactions
Oxytocics – enhances uterotonic effect

Pharmacodynamic properties
Causes contraction of the uterus and softening which decreases resistance of cervical tissue, depresses placental and uterine blood flow, but these actions are secondary to the main uterine stimulation

Fetal risk
ABORTIFACIENT

Breastfeeding
Not applicable

BP
Carboprost tromethamine

Proprietary
Hemabate Sterile Solution (Pharmacia Limited)

Group
Synthetic prostaglandin (F2α) and oxytocin

Uses/indications
Treatment of uterine atony in postpartum haemorrhage when ergometrine and oxytocin have already been used

Type of drug
POM

Presentation
Solution for injection

Dosage
1 mL contains carboprost tromethamine equivalent to carboprost 250 mcg
An initial dose of 250 mcg (1.0 mL) Hemabate as a deep IM injection
If necessary, further doses of 250 mcg may be administered at intervals of approximately 1.5 h
In severe cases the interval between doses may be reduced but it should not be less than 15 min
The total dose of Hemabate should not exceed 2 mg (8 doses)

Route of admin
Deep IM injection
Injection into the lower uterine segment to control severe haemorrhage

Contraindications
Hypersensitivity, acute pelvic inflammatory disease, known active cardiac, pulmonary, renal, or hepatic disease
NB: assessment of the benefit/risk ratio may be necessary

Side effects
Headache, flushing, hot flushes, chills, cough and body temperature increase

Interactions
Enhance the effect of other oxytocics

Pharmacodynamic properties
Stimulates the uterus to contract to promote homeostasis at the placental site and prevents further blood loss. Prostaglandins stimulate the smooth muscle to contract and inhibit the release of noradrenaline (norepinephrine)

Fetal risk
Not applicable

Breastfeeding
No evidence to say unsafe

BP
Mifepristone

Proprietary
Mifegyne® (Nordic Pharma Limited)

Group
Antiprogestogenic steroid

Uses/indications
Medical termination of developing intrauterine pregnancy
Softening and dilatation of the cervix prior to surgical termination of pregnancy during the first trimester
Preparation for the action of prostaglandin analogues in the termination of pregnancy for medical reasons *(beyond the first trimester)*
Induction for intrauterine death
where prostaglandin or oxytocin are contraindicated

Type of drug
POM

Presentation
Light yellow, cylindrical, bi-convex tablets

Dosage
Gestation up to 9 weeks: mifepristone 200 mg orally followed 1–3 days later by misoprostol 800 mcg vaginally; in women at more than 7 weeks' gestation (49–63 days), if the abortion has not occurred 4 h after misoprostol, a further dose of misoprostol 400 mcg may be given vaginally or orally
Gestation between 9 and 13 weeks: mifepristone 200 mg orally followed 36–48 h later by misoprostol

Continued

800 mcg vaginally followed if necessary by a maximum of 4 further doses at 3-hrly intervals of misoprostol 400 mcg vaginally or orally

Gestation between 13 and 24 weeks: mifepristone 200 mg orally followed 36–48 h later by misoprostol 800 mcg vaginally, then a maximum of 4 further doses at 3-hrly intervals of misoprostol 400 mcg orally

Route of admin
Oral

Contraindications
SHOULD NEVER be prescribed if: chronic adrenal failure, hypersensitivity, severe asthma (uncontrolled by therapy) or inherited porphyria

See SPC for specific contraindications in relation to the indications for use

Side effects
Headache, nausea, vomiting, diarrhoea, cramping, hypersensitivity: skin rashes, urticaria, erythroderma, erythema nodosum, toxic epidermal necrolysis, infection (endometritis, pelvic inflammatory disease), toxic shock, hypotension, malaise, hot flushes, dizziness, chills, fever, and uterine rupture

Interactions
Mifepristone is a CYP3A4 substrate and metabolized by CYP3A4 (a cytochrome P450 enzyme)

It is likely that ketoconazole, itraconazole, erythromycin and grapefruit juice may inhibit its metabolism (increasing serum levels of mifepristone) and toxicity also in the presence of CYP3A4 inhibitors and inducers

Rifampicin, dexamethasone, St John's wort and certain anticonvulsants (phenytoin, phenobarbital, carbamazepine) may induce mifepristone metabolism (lowering serum levels of mifepristone)

General anaesthetic may also enhance mifepristone toxicity

Pharmacodynamic properties
During pregnancy it sensitizes the myometrium to the contraction-inducing action of prostaglandin

Fetal risk
Data are too limited to determine teratogenicity, so if the method of termination fails further methods should be tried
NB: if the woman wishes to continue the pregnancy, close ultrasonographic follow-up is recommended

Breastfeeding
No data are available; therefore, should be avoided during breastfeeding

---

BP
Misoprostol

Proprietary
Cytotec® 200 mcg tablets (Pharmacia Limited)

Group
Synthetic prostaglandin

Uses/indications
Currently not licensed to induce medical abortion
Currently not licensed in postpartum haemorrhage
Used when oxytocin, ergometrine and carboprost are not available

Type of drug
Prostaglandin

Presentation
White to off-white hexagonal tablets

Dosage
See **MIFEPRISTONE** in relation to termination of pregnancy
PPH prevention – 600 mg orally (when oxytocic not available) (RCOG Greentop guideline 52, 2009)
PPH treatment – 1000 mg rectally (RCOG Greentop guideline 52, 2009)

Route of admin

Oral or vaginal

Contraindications

Women who are pregnant, or in whom pregnancy has not been excluded, or women planning a pregnancy as misoprostol increases uterine tone and contractions in pregnancy which may cause partial or complete expulsion of the products of conception. **However, used to induce medical abortion (unlicensed)** – see BNF for details

Side effects

Anaphylactic reaction, dizziness, headache, diarrhoea, abdominal pain, constipation, dyspepsia, flatulence, nausea, vomiting, rash, amniotic fluid embolism, abnormal uterine contractions, fetal death, incomplete abortion, premature birth, retained placenta, uterine rupture, uterine perforation, vaginal haemorrhage (including postmeno-pausal bleeding), intermenstrual bleeding, menstrual disorder, uterine cramping, menorrhagia, dysmenorrhoea, uterine haemorrhage, birth defects, chills and pyrexia

Interactions

In rare cases NSAIDs and misoprostol may cause a transaminase increase and peripheral oedema
Drug interaction studies have shown no significance in relation to and several NSAIDs, diclofenac, piroxicam, aspirin, naproxen or indometacin
Magnesium-containing antacids should be avoided during treatment with misoprostol as this may worsen the misoprostol-induced diarrhoea

Pharmacodynamic properties

Increases uterine tone and contractions in pregnancy which may cause partial or complete expulsion of the products of conception
An analogue of naturally occurring prostaglandin E_1, which promotes peptic ulcer healing and provides symptomatic relief

Protects the gastroduodenal mucosa by inhibiting basal, stimulated and nocturnal acid secretion, and by reducing the volume of gastric secretions, the proteolytic activity of the gastric fluid, and increasing bicarbonate and mucus secretion

Fetal risk
Associated with abortion, premature birth, and fetal death and birth defects

Breastfeeding
Should not be administered to nursing mothers as causes diarrhoea in infants

References and Recommended Reading

Baxter, K., 2011. Stockley's Drug Interaction Companion. Pharmaceutical Press, London.

Briggs, G., Freeman, R., Yaffe, S., 2008. Drugs in Pregnancy and Lactation: A Reference Guide to Fetal and Neonatal Risk, eighth ed. Lippincott Williams and Wilkins, Philadelphia.

Bubimschi, C., Weiner, C., 2010. Medication. In: James, D.K., Steer, P.J., Weiner, C.P., Gonik, B. (Eds.), High Risk Pregnancy: Management Options, fourth ed. Elsevier Saunders, London, pp 579–598.

Hofmeyr, G.J., Neilson, J.P., Alfreirevic, Z., Crowther, C., Duley, L., Gulmezoglu, M., Gyte, G.M., Hodnett, E.D., 2008. Pregnancy and Childbirth – A Cochrane Pocketbook. Wiley Cochrane Series, London.

Joint Formulary Committee, 2011. British National Formulary (BNF) 62. Pharmaceutical Press, London.

Jordan, S., 2010. Pharmacology for Midwives: The Evidence Base for Safe Practice, second ed. Palgrave Macmillan, Basingstoke.

Koren, G., 2007. Medication Safety in Pregnancy and Breastfeeding: The Evidence Based A–Z Clinician's Pocket Guide. McGraw-Hill, New York.

McGeown, P., 2011. Induction of labour and post-term pregnancy. In: Macdonald, S., Magill-Cuerden, J. (Eds.), Mayes' Midwifery, fourteenth ed. Baillière Tindall/Elsevier, Edinburgh, pp. 851–860.

National Institute of Health and Clinical Excellence (NICE), 2008. CG70 Induction of Labour Guideline. NICE, London.

Prostaglandins (PGE₂)

Royal College of Obstetricians and Gynaecologists (RCOG) 2011 The Care of Women Requesting Induced Abortion – Evidence-based Clinical Guideline No. 7. RCOG, London. Available: http://www.rcog.org.uk/files/rcog-corp/Abortion%20guideline_web_1.pdf [accessed 29 March 2012].

Rubin, P.C., Ramsey, M., 2007. Prescribing in Pregnancy, fourth ed. BMJ Books/Blackwell Publishing, Oxford.

Royal College of Obstetricians and Gynaecologists (RCOG), 2009. (revised 2011) Prevention and Management of Postpartum Haemorrhage. Greentop Guideline No. 52. RCOG, London. Available: http://www.rcog.org.uk/files/rcog-corp/GT52PostpartumHaemorrhage0411.pdf.

Sanchez-Ramos, L., Delke, I., 2010. Induction of labour and termination of previable pregnancy. In: James, D.K., Steer, P.J., Weiner, C.P., Gonik, B. (Eds.), High Risk Pregnancy: Management Options, fourth ed. Elsevier Saunders, London, pp. 1145–1168.

Schaefer, C., Peters, P.W.J., Miller, R.K. (Eds.), 2007. Drugs During Pregnancy and Lactation: Treatment Options and Risk Assessment, Academic Press/Elsevier, London.

SPC from the eMC, Cytotec® 200 mcg tablets, Pharmacia Limited, updated on the eMC 25/11/10.

SPC from the eMC, Gemeprost, Sanofi-Aventis, updated on the eMC 17/09/07.

SPC from the eMC, Haemabate Sterile Solution, Pfizer Limited, updated on the eMC 20/01/12.

SPC from the eMC, Mifegyne®, Nordic Pharma Ltd, updated on the eMC 14/07/11.

SPC from the eMC, Propess®, Ferring Pharmaceuticals Ltd, updated on the eMC 01/04/08.

SPC from the eMC, Prostin E2® vaginal gel 1mg/2 mg, Pharmacia Ltd, updated on the eMC 22/03/11.

SPC from the eMC, Prostin E2® vaginal tablets 3 mg, Pharmacia Ltd, updated on the eMC 23/03/11.

Tang, O., Gemzelle-Danielsson, K., Ho, P., 2007. Misoprostol: pharmokinetic profile, effects on the uterus and side-effects. Int J Gynaecol Obstet 99, S160–S167. Available: http://www.misoprostol.org/File/IJGO_pharm_Tang.pdf.

Volans, G., Wiseman, H., 2012. Drugs Handbook 2012–2013, thirty third ed. Palgrave Macmillan, Basingstoke.

23

Rectal Preparations – Laxatives and Haemorrhoid Preparations

Laxatives

These are medicines that loosen the bowel content and encourage evacuation. They are also known as aperients. Use of certain laxatives in pregnancy and the puerperium is generally considered safe. When both dietary and lifestyle changes or non-pharmacological preparations have failed or there are gastrointestinal or neurological conditions, there is a variety of pharmacological choices: bulk-forming agents, stimulant laxatives, stool softeners and osmotic preparations. Before prescribing laxatives it is important to ascertain that the patient is constipated and that the condition is not secondary to an underlying undiagnosed complaint.

Haemorrhoid Preparations

These come in the form of suppositories or topical creams and are made up of combinations of ingredients such as soothing compounds, e.g. local anaesthetic, and corticosteroids, e.g. hydrocortisone to alleviate the local inflammatory response; they may also contain mild astringents, vasoconstrictors and heparinoids to help relieve the haemorrhoid.

Anusol® – cream, ointment, suppositories – applied twice daily after a bowel movement, or one suppository twice daily – use neither for longer than 7 days

Scheriproct® – ointment or suppositories – apply twice daily for 5–7 days (3–4 times daily on first day if necessary), then once daily for a few days until symptoms have cleared, or one suppository daily after bowel movement for 5–7 days

Proctosedyl® – ointment or suppositories – apply twice daily after bowel movement, or insert one suppository twice daily after bowel movement – do not use either for longer than 7 days.

The student should be aware of:

- the effect of progesterone on the alimentary tract musculature
- factors predisposing to haemorrhoids
- the use of dietary and lifestyle measures to alleviate constipation and haemorrhoid discomfort
- regimes following surgical repair of third- or fourth-degree perineal trauma.

BP
Bisacodyl

Proprietary
Dulcolax® (Boehringer Ingelheim Ltd)

Group
Stimulant laxative

Uses/indications
Constipation

Type of drug
GSL

Presentation
Smooth white torpedo-shaped suppositories (P)
Gastroresistant tablets (GSL)

Dosage
Tablet 5–10 mg nocte, action over 10–12 h
One 10 mg suppository

Route of admin
Oral, P.R.

Contraindications
In patients with ileus, intestinal obstruction, acute abdominal conditions including appendicitis, acute inflammatory bowel diseases, and severe abdominal pain associated with nausea and vomiting, which may be indicative of the aforementioned severe conditions
In severe dehydration and in patients with known hypersensitivity to bisacodyl or any other component of the product
Should not be used when anal fissures or ulcerative proctitis with mucosal damage are present
Avoid use in children under 10 years
Should not be used for more than 5 consecutive days without investigating the cause of constipation

Side effects
Abdominal cramps; not for prolonged use as it can cause atonic non-functioning colon and hypokalaemia

Pharmacodynamic properties
Stimulation of the mucosa of the large intestine results in colonic peristalsis with promotion of accumulation of water, and electrolytes, in the colonic lumen. This results in a stimulation of defaecation, reduction of transit time and softening of the stool. Stimulation of the rectum causes increased motility and a feeling of rectal fullness

Interactions
If used with antacids and milk products the resistance of the coating of the tablets may be reduced resulting in dyspepsia and gastric irritation

Fetal risk
No data available but use only if the benefits outweigh the risks

Continued

Breastfeeding
Considered safe but use only if the benefits outweigh the risks

BP
Docusate sodium

Proprietary
Norgalax® (Norgine Ltd)

Group
Stimulant laxative

Uses/indications
Constipation

Type of drug
P

Presentation
Rectal gel (enema)

Dosage
Active ingredient docusate sodium 0.12 g in each 10 g microenema 1 micro-enema if required

Route of admin
P.R.

Contraindications
Haemorrhoids, anal fissures, rectocolitis, anal bleeding, abdominal pain, intestinal obstruction, nausea, vomiting, inflammatory bowel disease, ileus and known hypersensitivity to any of the ingredients

Side effects
Anal burning, rectal pain, rectal bleeding, diarrhoea, urticaria, hepatotoxicity

Pharmacodynamic properties
Used as a faecal softening agent; considered to ease constipation by increasing the penetration of fluid into the faeces thereby causing them to soften. Norgalax® is usually effective in 5–20 min

Interactions
May increase the resorption of medicines
Not to be used in combination with hepatotoxic agents

Fetal risk
Use only if the benefits outweigh the risks

Breastfeeding
Use only if the benefits outweigh the risks

BP
Senna

Proprietary
Senokot® tablets or syrup (Forum Health Products Ltd)

Group
Stimulant laxative

Uses/indications
Constipation

Type of drug
GSL

Presentation
Tablets (brown)

Dosage
Syrup – 2–4 5 mL spoonfuls at night (10–20 mL)
Tablets – 2–4 tablets nocte

Route of admin
Oral

Contraindications
Persistent abdominal symptoms
Avoid abuse as it can cause atonic non-functioning
colon and hypokalaemia

Side effects
Abdominal cramps, local irritation

Continued

Pharmacodynamic properties
The sugar moiety of sennosides is removed by bacteria in the large intestine, releasing the active anthrone fraction. This stimulates peristalsis via the submucosal and myenteric nerve plexuses. Sennosides act in 8–12 h

Interactions
No data available

Fetal risk
No reports of fetal or animal toxicity

Breastfeeding
Standardized preparations are considered safe

BP
Glycerin

Proprietary
Glycerol (Thornton & Ross Ltd)

Group
Stimulant laxative – rectal stimulant only

Uses/indications
Constipation

Type of drug
GSL

Presentation
Suppositories

Dosage
Adult: 4 g = one suppository

Route of admin
P.R.; the suppository should be dipped in water before insertion

Contraindications
Anal fissure, haemorrhoids

Side effects
Local irritation

Pharmacodynamic properties
Promotes peristalsis and evacuation of the lower bowel by virtue of its irritant action

Interactions
None known

Fetal risk
Should be avoided in pregnancy unless directed by a physician

Breastfeeding
Should be avoided during lactation unless directed by a physician

---

BP
Lactulose solution

Proprietary
Duphalac® (Abbott Healthcare Products Ltd)
Lactulose solution (non-proprietary, see BNF for details)

Group
Osmotic laxative

Uses/indications
Constipation

Type of drug
P

Presentation
A colourless to brownish yellow, clear or not more than slightly opalescent liquid

Dosage
15 mL b.d.

Route of admin
Oral

Continued

Contraindications
Galactosaemia, intestinal obstruction

Side effects
Flatulence, abdominal cramps and discomfort

Interactions
No data available

Pharmacodynamic properties

The active ingredient, lactulose, is metabolized in the colon by the sacchrolytic bacteria, producing low molecular weight organic acids, mainly lactic acid, that lower the pH of the colonic contents and promote the retention of water by an osmotic effect, thus increasing peristaltic activity

Fetal risk
No reports of teratogenicity or hazard to the fetus

Breastfeeding
Considered safe

BP
Liquid paraffin

Proprietary
Liquid Paraffin Oral Emulsion (non-proprietary, see BNF for details)

Group
Stool softener

Uses/indications
Temporary relief of constipation

Type of drug
P

Presentation
Liquid

Dosage
Adult: 10–30 mL when required

Route of admin
Oral

Contraindications
Children under 3 years of age

Side effects

Anal seepage of paraffin with consequent anal irritation after prolonged use

Granulomatous reaction caused by absorption of small quantities of liquid paraffin

Lipoid pneumonia (by accidental inhalation) may occur; therefore caution needed in patients with swallowing difficulty

Pharmacodynamic properties
Paraffin acts as a lubricant and penetrates and softens the stools

Interactions
May interfere with the absorption of fat-soluble vitamins

Fetal risk
Avoid during early pregnancy

Breastfeeding
Avoid during lactation

BP
Ispaghula husk

Proprietary
Fybogel® Orange (Forum Health Products Ltd)

Group
Bulk-forming laxatives

Continued

Uses/indications
Those requiring a high-fibre regime, e.g. relief of constipation, including constipation in pregnancy and the maintenance of regularity, management of bowel function in patients with a colostomy, ileostomy, haemorrhoids, anal fissure, chronic diarrhoea associated with diverticular disease, irritable bowel syndrome and ulcerative colitis

Type of drug
GSL

Presentation
Effervescent granules

Dosage
A unit dose (one sachet or two level 5 mL spoonfuls) contains 3.5 g ispaghula husk
One sachet or two level 5 mL spoonfuls morning and evening

Route of admin
Oral

Contraindications
Intestinal obstruction, faecal impaction and colonic atony

Side effects
Minor abdominal distension and flatulence

Interactions
None known

Pharmacodynamic properties
Ispaghula husk is able to absorb up to 40 times its own weight in water in vitro, and part of its activity can be attributed to its action as a simple bulking agent
Additionally, colonic bacteria are believed to use the hydrated material as a metabolic substrate, resulting in an increase in the bacterial cell mass and resulting in softening of the faeces

Fetal risk
May be used during pregnancy as the ispaghula husk is not absorbed from the gastrointestinal tract

Breastfeeding
May be used during lactation as the ispaghula husk is not absorbed from the gastrointestinal tract

References and Recommended Reading

Baxter, K., 2011. Stockley's Drug Interaction Companion. Pharmaceutical Press, London.

Briggs, G., Freeman, R., Yaffe, S., 2008. Drugs in Pregnancy and Lactation: A Reference Guide to Fetal and Neonatal Risk, eighth ed. Lippincott Williams and Wilkins, Philadelphia.

Bubimschi, C., Weiner, C., 2010. Medication. In: James, D.K., Steer, P.J., Weiner, C.P., Gonik, B. (Eds.), High Risk Pregnancy: Management Options, fourth ed. Elsevier Saunders, London, pp. 579–598.

Hofmeyr, G.J., Neilson, J.P., Alfreirevic, Z., Crowther, C., Duley, L., Gulmezoglu, M., Gyte, G.M., Hodnett, E.D. 2008. Pregnancy and Childbirth – A Cochrane Pocketbook. Wiley Cochrane Series, London.

Joint Formulary Committee, 2011. British National Formulary (BNF) 62. Pharmaceutical Press, London.

Jordan, S., Hegarty, B., 2010. Laxatives in pregnancy and the puerperium. In: Jordan, S. (Ed.), Pharmacology for Midwives: The Evidence Base for Safe Practice, second ed. Palgrave Macmillan, Basingstoke, pp. 272–283.

Koren, G., 2007. Medication Safety in Pregnancy and Breastfeeding: The Evidence Based A–Z Clinician's Pocket Guide. McGraw-Hill, New York.

Royal College of Obstetricians and Gynecologists (RCOG), 2007. The Management of Third and Fourth Degree Perineal Tears. Greentop Guideline No. 29. RCOG, London.

Rubin, P.C., Ramsey, M., 2007. Prescribing in Pregnancy, fourth ed. BMJ Books/Blackwell Publishing, Oxford.

Schaefer, C., Peters, P.W.J., Miller, R.K., 2007. Drugs During Pregnancy and Lactation: Treatment Options and Risk Assessment. Academic Press/Elsevier, London.

SPC from the eMC, Anusol®, suppositories, ointment and cream, McNeil Products Ltd, updated on the eMC 10/03/08, 10/03/08 and 07/10/10.

SPC from the eMC, DulcoLax® suppositories 10 mg and DulcoLax® tablets 5 mg, Boehringer Ingelheim Ltd Consumer Healthcare, updated on the eMC 05/08/11 and 06/06/11.

SPC from the eMC, Duphalac®, Abbott Healthcare Products Ltd, updated on the eMC 09/12/10.

SPC from the eMC, Fybogel® Orange, Forum Health Products Ltd, updated on the eMC 29/07/10.

SPC from the eMC, Glycerin Suppositories, Thornton & Ross Ltd, updated on the eMC 21/11/11.

SPC from the eMC, Liquid Paraffin BP, Thornton & Ross Ltd, updated on the eMC 21/11/11.

SPC from the eMC, Norgalax®, Norgine Ltd, updated on the eMC 13/12/10.

SPC from the eMC, Proctosedyl® ointment and suppositories, Sanofi-Aventis, updated on the eMC 18/09/07 and 24/09/07.

SPC from the eMC Scheriproct® ointment and suppositories, Bayer PLC, updated on, the eMC 08/12/06 and 08/12/06

SPC from the eMC, Senokot® tablets and syrup, Forum Health Products Ltd, updated on the eMC 02/08/10 and 02/08/10

Volans, G., Wiseman, H., 2012. Drugs Handbook 2012–2013, thirtythird ed.. Palgrave Macmillan, Basingstoke.

24

Vaccines

A vaccine is a suspension of dead or disabled organisms that, when ingested or injected, prevents, lessens or treats infections or disease. The most commonly used vaccines in midwifery are rubella (the single antigen vaccine is no longer available in the UK), hepatitis B and BCG vaccine. All women should be offered rubella-screening in early antenatal care to identify the risk of contracting rubella infection; this enables MMR (measles, mumps, rubella) vaccination to be offered following birth and before discharge.

Serological screening for hepatitis B virus should be offered to pregnant women so that effective postnatal intervention can be offered to infected women to decrease the risk of mother-to-child-transmission.

Vaccines are either live attenuated, which usually produce a durable immunity, although not necessarily as long-lasting as immunity resulting from natural infection, or inactivated; a series of injections of vaccine may be administered to produce an adequate antibody response.

The student should be aware of:

- detection of low levels of rubella antibodies in a client
- when it is appropriate to give vaccines in the postnatal period
- the sequlae of either vaccination or disease
- the possible side effects of vaccination.

BP
Rubella vaccine

Proprietary
Priorix® (GlaxoSmithKline UK)
(measles, mumps and rubella – MMR)

Group
Vaccine – live attenuated

Uses/indications
Vaccination where there are low levels of rubella
antibodies or none detected

Type of drug
POM

Presentation
Ampoules, powder and solvent for reconstitution

Dosage
Dependant on age of recipient

Route of admin
S.C. or IM

Contraindications
Pregnancy or the intention to become pregnant within
1 month; febrile patients
Systemic hypersensitivity to any component of the
vaccine or to neomycin
Extreme care if administered to individuals with egg allergy
Impaired immune function (however, recommend in
asymptomatic HIV infection)

Side effects
A mild form of the disease
Rash or swelling at the injection site (use a lesion-free
site if eczema)

Interactions
Possible interference from passive antibodies
Can be administered at the same time as the live varicella
vaccine (Varilix) but separate injection sites must be used

Priorix® cannot be given at the same time as other live attenuated vaccines; an interval of 4 weeks should be left between vaccinations

In individuals who have received human gammaglobulins or a blood transfusion, vaccination should be delayed for at least 3 months owing to the possibility of vaccine failure due to passively acquired mumps, measles and rubella antibodies

If being given primarily to achieve protection against rubella, the vaccine may be given within 3 months of the administration of an immunoglobulin preparation or a blood transfusion

If tuberculin testing is required, it should be carried out before, or simultaneously, as it has been reported that live measles (and possibly mumps) vaccine may cause a temporary depression of tuberculin skin sensitivity resulting in inconclusive results

If alcohol swabs are used to cleanse the skin, the alcohol must be allowed to evaporate as it may inactivate the vaccine

Pharmacodynamic properties
Induces active immunization against rubella virus infection

Fetal risk
Theoretical risk of teratogenicity and should therefore be avoided unless the need for vaccination outweighs the risk to the fetus

Breastfeeding
Available data suggest that breastfeeding is safe

BP
Hepatitis B vaccine

Proprietary
Engerix B® (GlaxoSmithKline UK)
HBvaxPRO® (Sanofi Pasteur MSD Ltd)

Continued

Group
Vaccine

Uses/indications
Active immunization against hepatitis B virus infection (HBV) caused by all known subtypes in non-immune subjects

Type of drug
POM

Presentation
Suspension for injection

Dosage
IM adult and child over 16 years: 3 doses of 20 mcg, the second 1 month and the third 6 months after the first dose
Neonate (except if born to hepatitis B surface antigen (HBsAg)-positive mother, see below) and child 1 month–16 years: 3 doses of 10 mcg
Neonate born to HBsAg-positive mother (see also notes above): 4 doses of 10 mcg, first dose at birth with hepatitis B immunoglobulin (HBIg) injection (separate site) the second 1 month, the third 2 months and the fourth 12 months after the first dose
NB: see manufacturers' information and BNF for other schedules and information on boosters

Route of admin
IM

Contraindications
Hypersensitivity

Side effects

Drowsiness, headache, nausea, vomiting, diarrhoea, abdominal pain, loss of appetite, pain and redness at injection site, fatigue, fever ($\geq$37.5°C), malaise, swelling at injection site, injection site reaction (such as induration), influenza-like illness, irritability, Apnoea in very premature infants ($\leq$28 weeks' gestation)

NB: due to the risk of apnoea, respiratory monitoring for 48–72h should be considered when administering the primary immunization series to infants born at ≤28 weeks of gestation and particularly those with a previous history of respiratory immaturity. The benefit of vaccination is high in this group of infants, so vaccination should not be withheld or delayed

Interactions

Administration of Engerix B® and a standard dose of HBIg does not result in lower anti-HBs antibody titres provided they are administered at separate injection sites
Can be given together with *Haemophilus influenzae* b, BCG, hepatitis A, polio, measles, mumps, rubella, diphtheria, tetanus and pertussis vaccines

Pharmacodynamic properties

Induces specific humoral antibodies against HBsAg (anti-HBs antibodies)
An anti-HBs antibody titre ≥10 IU/L correlates with protection to HBV infection

Fetal risk

No evidence available; use only if benefits outweigh possible risks

Breastfeeding

No evidence to say unsafe

BP
Bacille Calmette–Guérin vaccine

Proprietary
BCG Vaccine (SSI Denmark)

Group
Live attenuated vaccine

Uses/indications
Active immunization against tuberculosis

Continued

Type of drug
POM

Presentation
Powder and solvent for suspension for reconstitution as injection

Dosage
Adults and children aged 12 months and over: 0.1 mL of the reconstituted vaccine, infants under 12 months of age: a dose of 0.05 mL of the reconstituted vaccine

Route of admin
Intradermal

If alcohol swabs are used to cleanse the skin, the alcohol must be allowed to evaporate as it may inactivate the vaccine

Contraindications
Hypersensitivity; postponed if pyrexia or generalized skin infection; those receiving systemic corticosteroids or immunosuppressive treatment; not to be given to patients who are receiving antituberculous drugs

Side effects
The expected reaction to successful vaccination with BCG Vaccine SSI includes induration at the injection site followed by a local lesion that may ulcerate some weeks later and heal over some months later, leaving a small, flat scar

CAUTION: poor injection technique, overdose or an excessive response may result in a discharging ulcer

Interactions
May be given concurrently with inactivated or live vaccines, including combined measles, mumps and rubella vaccines

If other vaccines are administered at the same time, they should not be given into the same arm, or if not given at the same time an interval of not less than 4 weeks is recommended

Advised not to give further vaccination into the same arm used for BCG vaccination for 3 months due to the risk of regional lymphadenitis

Pharmacodynamic properties

Causes a cell-mediated immune response that confers a variable degree of protection to infection with *Mycobacterium tuberculosis*. The duration of immunity after BCG vaccination is not known, although it is considered that immunity reduces after 10 years

Fetal risk

BCG may be given during pregnancy if the benefit of vaccination outweighs the risk, or in populations considered at high risk of tuberculosis

Breastfeeding

BCG may be given during lactation if the benefit of vaccination outweighs the risk or in populations considered at high risk of Tuberculosis

References and Recommended Reading

Andrews, J.I., 2010. Hepatitis virus infections. In: James, D.K., Steer, P.J., Weiner, C.P., Gonik, B. (Eds.), High Risk Pregnancy: Management Options, fourth ed. Elsevier Saunders, London, pp. 469–478.

Baxter, K., 2011. Stockley's Drug Interaction Companion. Pharmaceutical Press, London.

Briggs, G., Freeman, R., Yaffe, S., 2008. Drugs in Pregnancy and Lactation: A Reference Guide to Fetal and Neonatal Risk, eighth ed. Lippincott Williams and Wilkins, Philadelphia.

Bubimschi, C., Weiner, C., 2010. Medication. In: James, D.K., Steer, P.J., Weiner, C.P., Gonik, B. (Eds.), High Risk Pregnancy: Management Options, fourth ed. Elsevier Saunders, London, pp. 579–598.

Hepatitis, B., Foundation UK. Education About Hepatitis B for Health and Social Care Professionals. Available: http://www.hepb.org.uk/information/resources/education_about_hepatitis_b_for_health_and_social_care_professionals [accessed 26 March 2012].

Hofmeyr, G.J., Neilson, J.P., Alfirevic, Z., Crowther, C., Duley, L., Gulmezoglu, M., Gyte, G.M., Hodnett, E.D., 2008. Pregnancy and Childbirth – A. Cochrane Pocketbook. Wiley Cochrane Series, London.

Joint Formulary Committee, 2011. British National Formulary (BNF) 62. Pharmaceutical Press, London.

Jordan, S., 2010. Pharmacology for Midwives: The Evidence Base for Safe Practice, second ed. Palgrave Macmillan, Basingstoke.

Koren, G., 2007. Medication Safety in Pregnancy and Breastfeeding: The Evidence Based A–Z Clinician's Pocket Guide. McGraw-Hill, New York.

Paediatric Formulary Committee, 2011. BNF for Children 2011–2012. Pharmaceutical Press, London.

Royal College of Obstetricians and Gynaecologists (RCOG), 2007. Clinical Greentop Guideline 13: Chickenpox in Pregnancy. RCOG, London.

Rubin, P.C., Ramsey, M., 2007. Prescribing in Pregnancy, fourth ed. BMJ Books/Blackwell Publishing, Oxford.

Schaefer, C., Peters, P.W.J., Miller, R.K. (Eds.), 2007. Drugs During Pregnancy and Lactation: Treatment Options and Risk Assessment, Academic Press/Elsevier, London.

SPC from the eMC, Engerix B®, GlaxoSmithKline UK, updated on 25/01/12.

SPC from the eMC, HBvaxPRO® (Sanofi Pasteur MSD Ltd), updated on 26/09/11.

SPC from the eMC, Human Hepatitis B Immunoglobulin, BPL (Bio Products Laboratory), updated on the eMC 15/01/09.

SPC from the eMC, Priorix®, GlaxoSmithKline UK, updated on the eMC 19/04/11.

Statens Serum Institute (SSI). BCG (bacille Calmette–Guérin) vaccine, available from health organizations or direct from ImmForm (SSI brand). Available: http://www.ssi.dk/English/Vaccines.aspx [accessed 8 February 2012].

Volans, G., Wiseman, H., 2012. Drugs Handbook 2012–2013, thirtythird ed. Palgrave Macmillan, Basingstoke.

UK National Screening Committee, UK Screening Portal. Available: http://www.screening.nhs.uk/ [accessed 26 March 2012].

25

Vitamins and Iron Preparations

Vitamins

Vitamins are factors in food necessary for growth and reproduction of living tissues. Some vitamins are fat soluble and others are water soluble. Those of interest to the midwife are vitamins C, B_{12}, K and folic acid, and are usually present in the diet.

Supplements of vitamins C and K are rare, but B_{12} and folic acid supplements are increasing. More recently, vitamin D has been in the spotlight with the re-emergence of neonatal rickets and reduced mineralization within the bones of children within certain populations. National Institute for Health and Clinical Excellence (NICE) guidelines were updated in 2008 to add advice for specific populations.

Other elements present in food are minerals.

The student should be aware of:

- the importance of good nutrition in women of childbearing age
- what is considered malnutrition by the World Health Organization (WHO)
- the prevalence of malnutrition in local populations
- the sequelae to mother and fetus of malnutrition
- the foods that are part of a well balanced healthy diet
- current recommendations for supplementation for specific populations (NICE, 2008).

Iron Preparations

Iron (Fe) is a metallic element and a constituent of the haemoglobin molecule that is necessary to carry oxygen around the body via the blood.

Vitamin C, and to a lesser extent folic acid, are involved in Fe absorption. In theory, the haemoglobin (Hb) concentration in the blood should increase by 2 g/100 mL, or 20 g/L, over 3–4 weeks of supplementation.

The student should be aware of:

- WHO guidelines for diagnosis of anaemia
- the aetiology of and predisposing factors for anaemia
- the physiology and pathophysiology of anaemia in pregnancy
- the appropriateness and effectiveness of Fe preparations, both in anaemia and routinely in pregnancy
- the different kinds of anaemia and their prognosis
- the dietary sources of Fe, vitamin C and folic acid
- the sequelae of anaemia in the antenatal, intranatal and postnatal periods.

NB: Because of the risk of anaphylactic reaction and cardiopulmonary collapse, Fe injections should be carried out under strict medical supervision. Resuscitation, defibrillation facilities and adrenaline (ephedrine) must be immediately available. It is also recommended that the course of oral Fe should be stopped 48 hours before the IM course.

A test dose is recommended prior to the first full administration.

Other Fe compounds

Pregaday® (UCB Pharma Ltd) – ferrous fumarate (100 mg Fe) and folic acid (350 mcg) tablets (brown) – one tablet daily (BNF, 2011).

BP
Ferrous sulphate

Proprietary
Ferrous sulphate (Goldshield Group UK Limited)
(non-proprietary, see BNF for details)

Group
Fe salts

Uses/indications
Iron deficiency anaemia

Type of drug
POM, GSL

Presentation
Tablets (white coated)

Dosage
One tablet 200 mg/day in prophylaxis or mild anaemia
2–3 tablets 400–600 mg/daily in therapeutic doses

Route of admin
Oral

Contraindications
Diverticulitis, inflammatory bowel disease, anaemias
other than iron deficiency, concurrent administration of
parenteral iron

Side effects
Nausea, gastric irritation, epigastric pain, diarrhoea or
constipation, iron overload, darkening of the stools

Interactions
Antacids – magnesium trisilicate reduces the absorption
of Fe
Antibiotics – absorption of antibiotics can be reduced in
the presence of Fe

Pharmacodynamic properties
Iron aids haemoglobin regeneration and the oxidative
processes in tissues

Continued

Fetal risk
No data available

Breastfeeding
Considered safe

BP
Iron dextran/sucrose compounds

Proprietary
CosmoFer® (Vitaline Pharmaceuticals UK Ltd) – 50 mg/mL iron as ferrous hydroxide with dextran
Venofer® (Vifor Pharma UK Ltd) – 20 mg/ml iron as ferrous hydroxide with sucrose

Group
Fe salts

Uses/indications
Failure of oral therapy, i.e. severe continuous blood loss, malabsorption

Type of drug
POM

Presentation
Ampoules

Dosage
Calculated according to client weight and iron deficiency – discontinue oral Fe 24 h prior to injection
An example for CosmoFer® is: 1.5 mg/kg body weight to a max 100 mg/day
Test dose of 25 mg to exclude anaphylactic reaction and remaining dose 60 min later

Route of admin
Deep IM (CosmoFer® only), slow IV or IV infusion
see manufacturer recommendations for dilutants (IV and infusion)

Contraindications
Liver and kidney disease (pyelonephritis), untreated urinary tract infection, early pregnancy, pre-existing

cardiac anomalies, existing asthma, allergic eczema or other atopic allergy should not be treated by IV injection; rheumatoid arthritis with active inflammation symptoms

Side effects
Anaphylactic reaction, pain at injection site, nausea, vomiting, dizziness, flushing, severe arrhythmias, theoretical risk of myocardial infarction, urine may turn black

Interactions
Chloramphenicol – may delay response to iron treatment; oral iron should not recommence until 5 days from last injection

Pharmacodynamic properties
Absorption from the injection site is rapid and complete, and therefore rapidly increases Fe stores for utilization as required

Fetal risk
May cause teratogenicity or abortion in early pregnancy; limit to second and third trimester recommended once risk/benefit assessed

Breastfeeding
No data, but manufacturers recommend avoidance

BP
Folic acid

Proprietary
Folic acid tablets BP (Actavis UK Ltd)
(non-proprietary, see BNF for details)

Group
Vitamins – B complex

Uses/indications
Folate-deficient megaloblastic anaemia, preconception until 12 weeks' gestation, prevention of neural tube defects

Continued

Type of drug
POM, GSL (doses must not exceed 500 mcg/day)

Presentation
Tablets, syrup

Dosage
Preconception or first 12 weeks of gestation: 400 mcg daily
In folate-deficiency anaemia: 5 mg/day for 4 months or
continued to term

Route of admin
Oral

Contraindications
Untreated pernicious anaemia or other cause of
cobalamin deficiency, including lifelong vegetarians

Side effects
No data available

Interactions
Antiepileptics – absorption of phenytoin or phenobarbital is reduced (plasma concentrations), increasing the
risk of seizures; therefore, advice should be taken on
supplementation
Antibacterials – chloramphenicol and co-trimoxazole
may interfere with folate metabolism

Fetal risk
No data available on overdosage

Breastfeeding
Actively excreted in breast milk; considered safe

BP
Vitamin B_{12} hydroxocobalamin

Proprietary
(non-proprietary, see BNF for details)

Group
Vitamins – B complex

Uses/indications
Very rare in pregnancy, pernicious anaemia, B_{12} deficiency

Type of drug
POM

Presentation
Ampoules

Dosage
1 mg, 3 times per week for two weeks; maintenance dose 1 mg every 3 months

Route of admin
Deep IM

Contraindications
Diagnosis of deficiency should be fully established

Side effects
Nausea, headaches, dizziness, fever, hypersensitivity and injection site reactions, hypokalaemia, and chromaturia

Interactions
Antiepileptics – reduced absorption of phenytoin or phenobarbital
Antibacterials – reduced response to chloramphenicol and co-trimoxazole

Fetal risk
Maternal B_{12} deficiency results in poor fetal outcome – there are no reports of high maternal dosage at *term* and maternal or fetal complications

Breastfeeding
Lack of B_{12} in the maternal diet can cause neonatal anaemia. Dietary supplements are recommended where deficiency is diagnosed

Continued

BP
Colecalciferol (vitamin D$_3$)

Proprietary
Accrete D3 (600 mg calcium and 400 IU colecalciferol (10 mcg) (Internis Pharmaceuticals Ltd)
Adcal-D3 (300 mg calcium and 200 IU colecalciferol (5 mcg) (ProStraken)

Group
Vitamins

Uses/indications
Calcium and vitamin D supplementation in at-risk groups

Type of drug
POM

Presentation
Film-coated tablet/caplet – ochre/pale orange respectively

Dosage
600 IU per day (NICE, 2008: CG62 and PH11)

Route of admin
Oral

Contraindications
Hypercalcaemia, hypercalciuria, renal disease, hypersensitivity to active substances, immobility

Side effects
Hypercalcaemia, hypercalciuria, abdominal pain, constipation, diarrhoea, nausea, flatulence, skin rashes

Interactions
Thiazide diuretics – reduced excretion of calcium
Tetracycline: calcium salts can interfere with tetracycline absorption
Cardiac glycosides – increased toxicity of cardiac glycosides, e.g. digitalis, oxalic acid (spinach, rhubarb and sorrel) and phytic acid (cereals) can reduce calcium absorption

Pharmacodynamic properties
Increases calcium absorption from intestine; counteracts parathyroid hormone production when calcium levels are depleted, colecalciferol converted to 25-hydroxy-colecalciferol in liver and 1,25-hydroxycolecalciferol in kidney, which increases calcium absorption

Fetal risk
Vitamin D: animal studies – toxicity at high doses
Calcium and vitamin D: prolonged hypercalcaemia may lead to impaired physical and mental development, supraventricular aortic stenosis and retinopathy

Breastfeeding
Calcium and vitamin D pass via breast milk and this needs to be considered should supplements be required

References and Recommended Reading

Baxter, K., 2011. Stockley's Drug Interaction Companion. Pharmaceutical Press, London.

Briggs, G., Freeman, R., Yaffe, S., 2008. Drugs in Pregnancy and Lactation: A Reference Guide to Fetal and Neonatal Risk, eigth ed. Lippincott Williams and Wilkins, Philadelphia.

Bubimschi, C., Weiner, C., 2010. Medication. In: James, D.K., Steer, P.J., Weiner, C.P., Gonik, B. (Eds.), High Risk Pregnancy: Management Options, fourth ed. Elsevier Saunders, London, pp. 579–598.

Joint Formulary Committee, 2011. British National Formulary (BNF) 62. Pharmaceutical Press, London.

Jordan, S., 2010. Nutritional supplements in pregnancy. In: Jordan, S. (Ed.), Pharmacology for Midwives: The Evidence Base for Safe Practice, second ed. Palgrave Macmillan, Basingstoke, pp. 249–262.

Koren, G., 2007. Medication Safety in Pregnancy and Breastfeeding: The Evidence Based A–Z Clinician's Pocket Guide. McGraw-Hill, New York.

Macdonald, S., Magill-Cuerden, J., 2011. Mayes' Midwifery, fourteen ed. Baillière Tindall/Elsevier, Edinburgh.

National Institute for Health and Clinical Excellence (NICE), 2008. CG62: Antenatal Care: Routine Care for the Healthy Pregnant Woman. NICE, London.

National Institute for Health and Clinical Excellence (NICE), 2008. Public Health Guidance PH11: Improving the Nutrition of Pregnant and Breast Feeding Mothers and Children in Low-income Households. NICE, London.

Pregaday® tablets (100 mg iron and 350 mcg folic acid), UCB Pharma, updated in BNF 62, 2011.

Rubin, P.C., Ramsey, M., 2007. Prescribing in Pregnancy, fourth ed. BMJ Books/Blackwell Publishing, Oxford.

Schaefer, C., Peters, P.W.J., Miller, R.K. (Eds.), 2007. Drugs During Pregnancy and Lactation: Treatment Options and Risk Assessment, Academic Press/Elsevier, London.

SPC from the eMC, Accrete D3® tablets, Internis Pharmaceuticals Ltd, updated on the eMC 7/12/11.

SPC from the eMC, Adcal-D3® caplets, ProStraken, updated on the eMC 1/9/11.

SPC from the eMC, CosmoFer® injection, Vitaline Pharma UK, updated on the eMC 27/1/10.

SPC from the eMC, Ferrous Sulphate 200 mg tablets, Goldshield Group Ltd, updated on the eMC 15/11/10.

SPC from the eMC, Folic Acid tablets BP 5 mg, Actavis UK Ltd, updated on the eMC 15/12/10.

SPC from the eMC, Venofer® injection, Vifor Pharma UK Ltd, updated on the eMC 30/3/11.

Volans, G., Wiseman, H., 2012. Drugs Handbook 2012–2013, thirty third ed. Palgrave Macmillan, Basingstoke.

World Health Organization, 2011. WHO, Nutrition Experts Take Action on Malnutrition. Available: http://www.who.int/nutrition/press note_action_on_malnutrition/en/ [accessed 31 March 2012].

Further Reading

The Cochrane Library. Available: http://www.thecochranelibrary.com/ [accessed 30 March 2012] (various evidence-based information reviews on supplements in pregnancy and postnatal periods).

Drug Calculations

The NMC Standards for Medicines Management state:

> 'Some drug administrations can require complex calculations to ensure that the correct volume or quantity of medication is administered. In these situations, it is good practice for a second practitioner (a registered professional) to check the calculation independently in order to minimise the risk of error. The use of calculators to determine the volume or quantity of medication should not act as a substitute for arithmetical knowledge or skill'

(NMC, 2007, updated 2010, Section 4: Standard 8, p38)

The student should be aware of:

- the NMC publications – The Code (NMC, 2008) and Standards for Medicines Management (NMC, 2007, updated 2010)
- local NHS Trust guidelines for medicines management relating to administration
- drug calculation formulas used within their clinical practice (adult and neonatal) and competence in manipulation of numerical values within these formulas.

The Basic Formula

$$\frac{\text{required strength}}{\text{available strength}} \times \text{quantity preparation is supplied in}$$

or

$$\frac{\text{what you want}}{\text{what you've got}} \times \text{IT (the preparation)}$$

e.g. ampicillin elixir 125 mg/mL – the prescription says 100 mg, therefore:

$$\frac{100}{125} \times 5 = 4 \text{ mL}$$

e.g. benzyl penicillin 600 mg/5 ml the prescription says 200 mg, therefore:

$$\frac{200}{600} \times 5 = 1.66 \text{ mL}$$

For Rates of Infusion

$$\text{Flow rate in mL/h} = \frac{\text{Volume of fluid (mL)}}{\text{Time to infuse (h)}}$$

$$\text{e.g. Flow rate} = \frac{500}{8} = 62.5 = 63 \text{ mL/h}$$

If the infusion is to run over minutes then divide by the number of minutes to run:

$$\text{Flow rate in drops / min} = \frac{\text{mL to be infused}}{\text{hrs to be delivered}} \times \frac{\text{no. of drops per mL}}{\text{time in minutes (60)}}$$

e.g. 1 L fluid over 12 h, using a burette (60 drops/mL):

$$\text{Flow rate} = \frac{1000}{12} \times \frac{60}{60} = 83 \text{ drops/min}$$

e.g. 450 mL blood over 3 h using a blood-giving set (15 drops/mL):

$$\text{Flow rate} = \frac{450}{3} \times \frac{15}{60} = 37.5 = 38 \text{ drops/min}$$

An alternative mode of calculation that may be used utilizes a drop rate denominator (DRD):

$$\text{DRD} = \frac{\text{No. of drops per mL delivered by administration set (drop factor)}}{\text{No. of minutes in 1 h (i.e. 60 min)}}$$

60 drops per mL = 1 DRD
20 drops per mL = 3 DRD
15 drops per mL = 4 DRD
12 drops per mL= 5 DRD
10 drops per mL = 6 DRD

e.g. 450 mL blood over 3 h using a blood-giving set (15 drops/mL):

$$\text{Flow rate} = \frac{450}{3} = 150$$

$$\text{Then , } 150/(\text{DRD}) = \frac{150}{4} = 37.5 = 38 \text{ drops per min}$$

Neonatal Calculation

Students should also be able to use a formula that requires doses to be calculated from measures of weight.

e.g. neonatal paracetamol suspension – dose 10 mg/kg. So, for an infant weighing 3 kg (or 3000 g), the dose required would be 30 mg. Paracetamol suspension is 120 mg in 5 mL:

$$\frac{\text{what you want}}{\text{what you've got}} \times \text{IT (the preparation)}$$

$$\text{i.e. } \frac{30 \text{ mg}}{120 \text{ mg}} \times 5 \text{ mL} = 1.25 \text{ mL}$$

References

Lapham, R., Agar, H., 2009. Drug Calculations for Nurses – A Step-by-step Approach, third ed. Hodder Arnold, London.

Nursing and Midwifery Council (NMC), 2007. updated 2010 Standards for Medicines Management. NMC, London.

Nursing and Midwifery Council (NMC), 2008. The Code: Standards of Conduct, Performance and Ethics for Nurses and Midwives. NMC, London.

Wright, K., 2011. Drug Calculations for Nurses: Context for Practice. Palgrave McMillan, Basingstoke.

INDEX